I0489760

Visceral Leishmaniasis

Signalling Approaches ——————

"The roots of Education are bitter,
but the fruit is sweet"

--- Aristotle

Visceral Leishmaniasis

Signalling Approaches ─────────

Dr. Debjani Das (Ghosh), M.Sc., Ph.D., B.Ed.

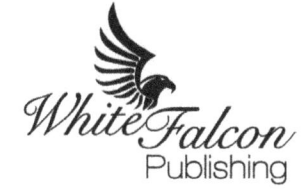

White Falcon
Publishing

Visceral Leishmaniasis: Signalling Approaches
Dr. Debjani Das (Ghosh)

www.whitefalconpublishing.com

All rights reserved
First Edition, 2019
© Dr. Debjani Das (Ghosh), 2019
Cover design © White Falcon Publishing, 2019
Cover image © Shutterstock.com

No part of this publication may be reproduced, or stored
in a retrieval system, or transmitted in any form by means
of electronic, mechanical, photocopying or otherwise,
without prior written permission from the author.

Requests for permission should be addressed to
Dr. Debjani Das (Ghosh)

ISBN - 978-93-88459-88-4

DEDICATED
TO

MY PARENTS AND HUSBAND

ACKNOWLEDGEMENTS

I would like to express my sincerest reverence to Dr. Prasanta Chakraborty, Indian Institute of Chemical Biology (IICB) and Dr. Mukul Kumar Basu, Ex-Emeritus Scientist (Ex-Director Grade Scientist and Ex-Head Biomembrane Division), IICB for their constant inspiration, constructive criticism and overall guidance and supervision in successful completion of this work.

I am extremely grateful to Professor Samir Bhattacharya, Ex-Director, Indian Institute of Chemical Biology for his invaluable help and support.

I am also thankful to Indian Council of Medical Research (ICMR) and Lady Tata Memorial Trust for providing financial assistance in carrying out this work.

I am indebted to, Drs., H.K. Mazumdar, P.K. Das, (Mrs.) N. Ali, S. Roy, M. Bagchi, R. K, Bhadra, S. Adhya, E. Ali, (Mrs.) N. Ghosal, S. Bandopadhyay, N.Das, and U. Dasgupta who have long been my valued advisers.

My heartiest gratitude is for my parents for their constant inspiration, for bearing all the troubles and for motivating me throughout the tenure of my research work.

Last but not the least, my husband, Dr. Narayan Chandra Das, Associate Professor, Scottish Church College, Kolkata deserves special acknowledgement for his constant active help, valuable suggestions and constructive criticism in successful completion of this work.

Dr. Debjani Das (Ghosh)

ABBREVIATIONS

DNA	Deoxyribonucleic acid
RE	Reticuloendothelial
TCA	Tricarboxylic acid
ATP	Adenosine triphosphate
AMP	Adenosine monophosphate
RBC	Red Blood Corpuscles
TNF-α	Tumor necrosis factor-α
IFN-γ	Interferon-γ
ELISA	Enzyme linked Immuno Sorbent Assay
lgG	lmmunoglobulin-G
RNA	Ribonucleic acid
RER	Rough endoplasmic reticulum
MHC	Major histocompatibility complex
AGE	Advanced glycosylation end (products)
IL	Interleukin
LDL	Low density lipoprotein
NADPH	Nicotinamide adenine dinucleotide phosphate (reduced)
PBS	Phosphate Buffered Saline
EDTA	Ethyline diamine tetraacetic acid
DMSO	Dimethyl sulfoxide
EGTA	Ethylene glycol-bis (β-aminoethyl Ether) - N, N, N', N'-tetracetic acid
HEPES	(4-(2-hydroxyethyl)- 1- piperazineethane sulphonic acid
PMSF	Phenyl methyl sulphonyl fluoride
DMEM	Dulbecco's Modified Eagle Medium
DAG	Diacyl glycerol
PS	Phosphatidyl serine
DPH	Diphenyl hexatriene

CONTENTS

INTRODUCTION

1

1.1 The parasite: *Leishmania donovani*

1.1.1 History of the parasite identity

In the annual report of the Inspector General of Civil Hospitals, 1872, (1) it was the first to mention about the topic kala-azar. In 1899, Ross identified it as 'Kala-azar'. In 1900, Sir William Boog Leishman, a Scottish Scientist discovered *L.donovani* in spleen smears of a soldier at Dum-Dum, India, who died of a fever. The disease was then termed locally as Dum-Dum fever. In 1903, Leishman published his observation; in the same year Charles Donovan, a Madras based Scientist, found the same parasite in spleen biopsy. The parasite was named *Leishmania donovani* as a new genus and species paying honours to these men, as did the common name of the amastigote forms, Leishman-Donovan (L-D) bodies, The Indian Kala-azar commission (1931 to 1934) demonstrated the transmission of *Leishmania donovani* by *Phlebotomus* spp.(1).

1.1.2 *Leishmania donovani*: Basic Biology

A member of the Trypanosomatid protozoa Leishmanias are heteroxenous. The intermediate hosts and vectors are sand flies (Family: Psychodidae; subfamily: Phlebotominae). Varied species of genus *Leishmania* with a common morphologic and ultrastructural character are the causative agent of a wide variety of Leishmaniasis. They are probably evolved from early Trypanosomatids (2).

1.1.2.1 Phylogenetic status

Several schemes of classification have been proposed keeping in view the difficulty in species identification within genus.

The given phylogenetic status is based on Hausmaun K, Hülsmann N, Protozoology, New York: Thieme Medical Publishers, Inc., 1996 (10).

Phylum	-	Euglenozoa
Subphylum	-	Kinetoplasta
Class	-	Trypanosomatidea
Family	-	Trypanosomatidae
Order	-	Trypanosomatida
Genus	-	*Leishmania*
Species	-	*donovani*

1.1.2.2 Morphology of the parasite

The parasite exists in two forms —

| Amastigote | - | Aflagellated form inside the vertebrate host (Fig. 1A-1) |
| Promastigote | - | Flagellated form, inside the vector, sandfly or in artificial cultures (Fig. 1A-2) |

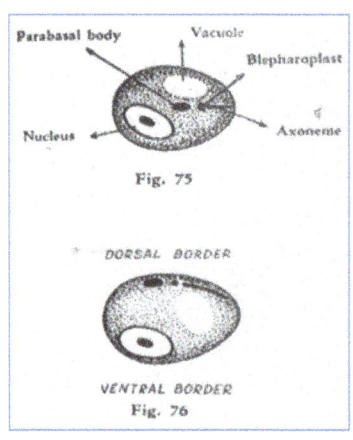

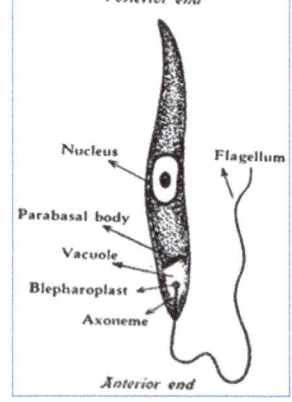

FIG. 1A-1: Amastigote   FIG 1A-2: Promastigote

(Courtesy, K.D.Chatterjee, 1975)

Amastigote

It is a non-motile form. Usually 2-5 μm wide, spheroid to ovoid in shape (often called Leishman-Donovan bodies). This is a hardy stage (3). It is among the smallest, nucleated cells known. In stained condition, only the large nucleus and very large kinetoplast can be seen and vacuolated cytoplasm appears. Under light microscope, a central nucleus and an exceptionally short axoneme within the cytoplasm are visible. The position of the rod-shaped kinetoplast is terminal or subterminal (4-9) and sometimes a basal body is found from which the flagellum arises (10, 11).

Promastigote

It is a free-swimming, flagellated form with single flagellum at the anterior end. The promastigotes which are fully developed are long, slender, spindle-shaped, varying in size, 15 – 20μm in length and 1 – 2 μm in breadth. The flagellum is often large or as long as the whole cell body. The cell consists of nucleus, cytoplasm, Kinetoplast mitochondria, etc. (2, 4 –7). Kinetoplast is present at the terminal or sub-terminal end (2, 4, 5, 12).

1.1.2.3 Parasite's ultrastructure

Electron microscopic studies revealed almost similar cellular organization in both the forms (5, 6, 13) (Fig.1A).

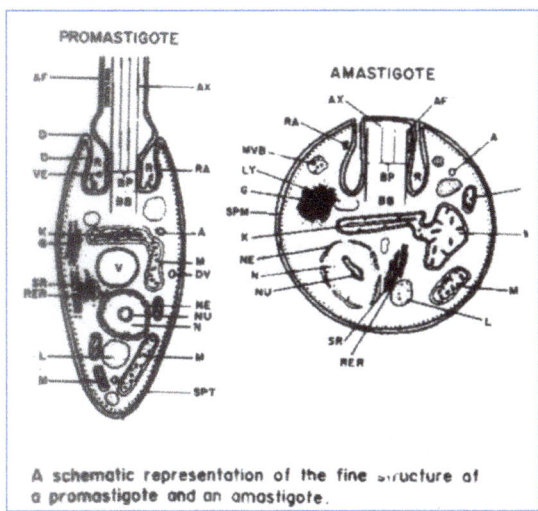

FIG. 1A: **A**-Acanthosome; **AF**-accessory filament; **Ax**-axoneme; **BB**-basal body; **BP**-basal plage; **D**-desmosome; **DV**-dense inclusion vesicle; **G**-lipid; **Ly**-lysosome; **M**-Mitochondria; **MVB**-multi vesiculate body; **MT**-subpelicular microtubules; **N**-nucleus; **NE**-nuclear envelop; **NU**-Nucleolus; **R**-reservoir; **RA**-reservoir associated microtubule; **RER**-rough endoplasmic reticulum; **SC**-surface coat; **SPM**-subpellicular micromolecules; **SR**-smooth reticulum; **V**-vacuole associated with nucleus; **VE**-vesicle

Nucleus — Ovoid or spheroid nucleus is located centrally in both the forms. In amastigotes, it is less than 1 μm in diameter.

Plasma membrane — It is invaginated and forms a reservoir called flagellar reservoir at the anterior end of *Leishmania*. In amastigotes, flagellum is confined within the reservoir but in promastigotes it is extended beyond the opening of the reservoir.

Microtubular system — This system has a significance in *Leishmania* as it provides rigidity and confirmation of the cell (5). Major functional microtubules are: subpellicular flagellar mitotic and reservoir associated microtubule.

Mitochondria — Mitochondrion (single) branches into many segments.

Kinetoplast complex — Tangentially or right-angled to the nucleus lies the kinetoplast. The kinetoplast is shown to be a specialised, disc-shaped, DNA containing organelle within highly extended convoluted mitochondrion (10). The root of the flagellum is represented by Axonemes (rhizoplast) which is a delicate filament extending from the margin of the body till the kinetoplast. Kinetoplast DNA (kDNA) is organised into a network of linked circles, quite unlike the organization of DNA in a chromosome (14). There are upto 20,000 tiny circles (minicircles) and 20 to 50 larger circles (maxicircles) in the kinetoplast network. Both maxi- and minicircles are joined to form a single structural unit. Although the function of minicircles is unknown, maxicircles are functionally analogues to mitochondrial DNAs (15).

Cell Division — Ultra structure reveals that during cell division, the division of the basal body, flagellum, flagellar reservoir, kinetoplast and nucleus, precedes that of the cell (2, 5, 7, 12).

1.1.2.4 Life cycle

The life cycle of *Leishmania* is completed through a definitive host, a mammal (including man) and an intermediate host, the phlebotomine fly (Fig.1B).

From a motile, extracellular inhabitant of the lumen of insect gut to a non-motile intracellular parasite of vetebrate's macrophage, the organism is repeatedly transformed to and fro. This oscillating circle is a must during the profound biological changes.

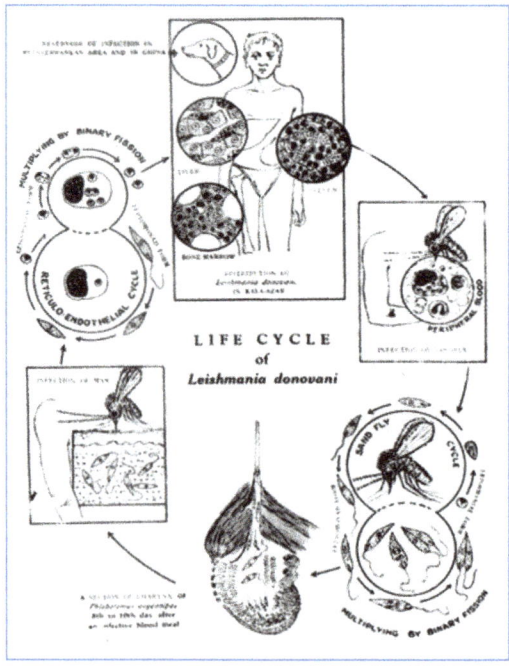

FIG. 1B: Life Cycle of Leishmania donovani

(Courtesy, K.D.Chatterjee, 1975)

Stage in invertebrate vector

Soon after lodging inside the fly gut, *Leishmania* differentiates from amastigote to slender promastigote and quickly blocks the gut of the insect. From the gut (hind gut or mid gut of the fly), the parasite moves towards oesophagus, then to the pharynx. From the pharynx, it migrates to the proboscis. Promastigotes attach strongly to the cuticle of the pharynx. In the proboscis, a few highly active promastigotes can be found. When the proboscis is invaded, the sandfly becomes infective and bites the next man or another host. Depending upon the species of *Leishmania* and also the sandfly, from the uptake of amastigotes to delivery of promastigotes, time taken is 6-25 days (10).

Stage in vertebrate vector

Once inside the mammalian host, they parasitize a macrophage, lodge and multiply within long lived phagolysosome like parasitophorous vacuoles (PV) (16). Parasites multiply by binary fission and thus eventually kill the host cell. The parasites are then engulfed by other macrophages. Escaping dead macrophages, they eventually burst out to invade the new macrophages, which they also kill (17). By this means they severely damage the RE system (10), a system that plays a critical role in the host defense. The parasitised macrophages with blood meal are then ingested by sandfly and are ruptured and amastigotes are released in the gut and transform into promastigotes and new cycle starts (13).

Various routes of parasites

During visceral infection, after entering the host, the parasites invade cells of RE system where they reside and multiply. The proliferation of infection occurs in the tissues of viscera, including spleen, liver, mesenteric lymph nodes, intestine and bone marrow in case of *L. donovani* infection (10).

1.1.3 Parasite cell biology

Throughout their digenetic life cycle, *Leishmania* resides in the hydrolytic environment of the host. Interactions between the host and the parasite (all the physiologic and biochemical) occur across the surface membrane of the parasites or at the beginning of it, thus this must play a crucial role in survival and replication of the parasite within the infected host (6).

1.1.3.1 Charge characteristics

Both membrane phospholipids (Phosphate groups) and membrane carbohydrate contents are negatively charged, thus *Leishmania* promastigotes possess a net negative surface charge (6, 18-20).

1.1.3.2 Surface carbohydrates

By random cellular agglutination with various lectins, the presence of uniform distribution of specific carbohydrate ligands on the surface of *Leishmania* has been demonstrated (6, 19-23). D-mannose/glucose, D-galactose, N-acetylgalactosamine, N-acetyl glucosamine, L-fucose are among the very common carbohydrates identified.

The *Leishmania* parasites have adapted not only to survive but to proliferate largely due to protection conferred by unique glycoconjugates on parasite cell surface or secreted (24).

1.1.3.3 Membrane Proteins

In *L. donovani* promastigotes, 23 surface membrane proteins ranging in the molecular weight from $< 14.5 \times 10^3$ to $> 2.8 \times 10^5$ have been identified (25), all of which are mannose-containing glycoproteins.

1.1.3.4 Membrane lipids

About 60% and 30% of total neutral lipids present on the Leishmanial membrane (18) are composed of sterols and diglycerides respectively (26). Phospholipid content is about 70% of the total surface lipid of which phosphatidyl ethanolamine is the major one (6).

1.1.3.5 Cell Surface Enzymes

L.donovani surface membrane contains acid phosphatase, a mannose containing glycoprotein (27, 28). Alongwith 3' and 5' nucleotidase, (6, 18, 29), at the external face, which seems to fulfill a nutritional role. Mg^{+2}-ATPase and adenylatecyclase activities are also shown in the surface membrane. Numerous control and signal recognition processes are attenuated by cyclic AMP (6). *L.donovani* surface membrane is also associated with three distinct lipolytic enzymes, a thermolabile phospholipase-C, a heat stable phospholipase - A_2 and an uncommon phospholipase- A_1, which may have a role in altering or restructuring the phospholipid structure in its vicinity or in changing the composition of host cell phagolysosomal membrane. Membrane fluidity and its recycling to and fro the cellular compartment may be affected by these properties (6, 18).

1.1.3.6 Surface antigen

Surface bound antigens are expressed by *Leishmania* and which may play a role in virulency of the pathogens (30, 31). Schematic presentation of glycoproteins (gp 63) and lipophosphoglycan (LPG) of *Leishmania* is shown in (Fig.1C).

1.1.4 Metabolism of *Leishmania*

The uptake of sugar: hexoses; amino acids: methionine and proline; base purines by several species of Leishmanial promastigotes, is performed by carrier-mediated pathways. Presence of highly active and both 5' and 3' nucleotidase (6, 18, 29) transport activities in plasma membrane indicate that the parasites depend on exogeneous nucleotides as unable to synthesize it *de novo* (2,6,18). In both stages of *Leishmania*, Glycolytic and TCA cycle enzymes are found. Gluconeogenesis mediated by transaminases, which converts certain amino acids into TCA cycle intermediates, is very high in *Leishmania* sp. (2, 6, 18, 29). Cyclopropane fatty acids and ergosterols are found to be common fatty acids and sterols in *Leishmania* (2).

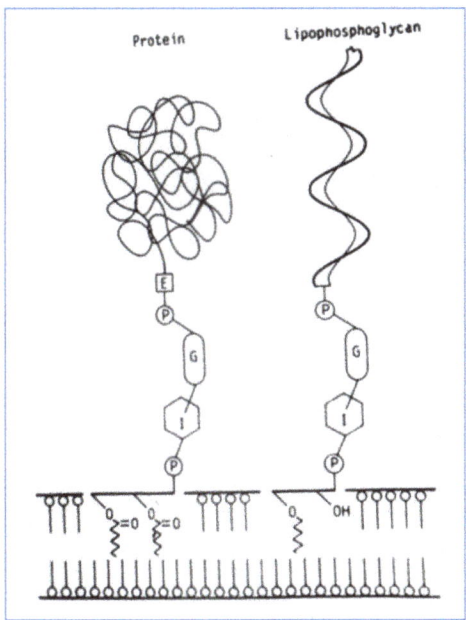

FIG.1C: Schematic presentation of glycoproteins (gp63) and Lipophosphoglycan (LPG)

1.1.5 The Disease Leishmaniasis

On the basis of infection the disease includes visceral, cutaneous and mucosal Leishmaniasis (32). The wide variety of forms of the disease is caused by about 21 different species of *Leishmania* (Table 1A). The intermediate hosts and vectors of *Leishmania* are over 600 species of sandflies divided into five Genera: *Phlebotomus, Sergentomyia* in the Old World and *Lutzomyia, Brumptomyia, Warileya* in the New World (10).

TABLE-1A: Species and Subspecies of *Leishmania*

Parasite	Locality
Subgenus *Leishmania* (Ross, 1903)	
L.donovani phenetic complex *L.donovani* (Laveran and Mesnil, 1903) *L.archibaldi* (Castellani and Chalmers, 1919) *L.infantum* phenetic complex	India, China, Bangladesh Sudan, Ethiopia
L.infantum (Nicolle, 1908)	North central Asia, northwest China, Middle East, southern Europe, northwest Africa
L.chagasi (Cunha and Chagas,1937) *L.tropica* phenetic complex *L.tropica* (Wright, 1903)	South and Central America Urban areas of Middle East and India
L.killicki (Rioux,Lanotte, Pratlong, 1986)	Tunisia
L.major phenetic complex *L.major*	Africa, Middle East, Soviet Asia

TABLE 1A: *Cont.*

Parasite	Locality
Subgenus *Leishmania* (Ross, 1903)	
L.gerbilli phenetic complex *L.gerbilli* (Wang,Qu,and Guan, 1973) *L. arabica* phenetic complex *L.arabica* (Peters,Elbihari, and Evans, 1986) *L.aethiopica* phenetic complex *L.aethiopica* (Bray, Ashford, and Bray, 1973) *L.mexicana* phenetic complex *L.mexicana* (Biagi, 1953) *L.amazonensis* (Lainson and Shaw, 1972) *L.venezuelensis* (Bonfante-Garrido, 1980) *L.enrietti* phenetic complex *L.enrietti* (Muniz and Medina, 1948) *L.hertigi* phenetic complex *L.hertigi* (Herrer, 1971) *L.deanei* (Lainson and Shaw, 1977)	China, Mongolia Saudi Arabia Ethiopia, Kenya Mexico, Belize, Guatemala, South central United States Amazon Basin, Brazil Venezuela Brazil Panama, Costa Rica Brazil
Subgenus Viannia (Lainson and Shaw, 1987)	
L.brazilliensis phenetic complex *L.brazilliensis* (Viannia, 1911) *L.peruviana* (Velez, 1913) *L.guyanensis* phenetic complex *L.guyanensis* (Floch, 1954) *L.panamensis* (Lainson and Shaw, 1972)	Brazil Western Andes French Guiana, Guyana, Surinam Panama, Costa Rica

Different forms of Leishmaniasis

The disease Leishmaniasis can be classified as:

1.1.5.1 Visceral Leishmaniasis (VL) or Kala-azar

The causative species of visceral Leishmaniasis are *L.donovani donovani, L.donovani infantum, L. donovani tropica* (Old-world) and *L. donovani chagasi, L. donovani amazonensis* (New world) (2). Worldwide distribution of visceral Leishmaniasis is shown in Fig.1D. This may be classified as:

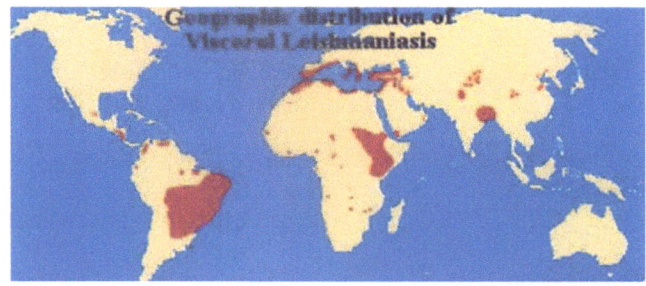

FIG. 1D: Worldwide distribution of Visceral Leishmaniasis.
Marked in red shows the areas affected by Visceral Leishmaniasis

(Courtesy, Google web page)

Endemic VL - This especially affects children (1-4 years) in the S-W Asia, China, S-America and Mediterranean area. Common symptoms are fever, malaria, weight loss, anorexia, anaemia, skin darkening and spleen enlargement.

Sporadic VL - This affects non-indigenous people entering an epidemic area and is marked by fever, 3 weeks to 2 years after exposure.

Epidemic VL - All ages are susceptible to this except old enough to have been affected during a previous epidemic.

It is further subdivided on the basis of reservoir as African Kala-azar (rodent reservoir), Mediterranean kala-azar (canine reservoir) and Indian kala-azar (human reservoir) (10).

Clinical manifestations of enlargement and marked alterations in function of liver and spleen (hepatosplenomegaly), bone marrow, lymph nodes, hypergammaglobulinemia with hypoalbuminaemia, hyperplasia, severe anaemia and emaciation (33), changes in hair color, and edema are recorded (2) (Fig. 1 $E_{i\text{-}iii}$).

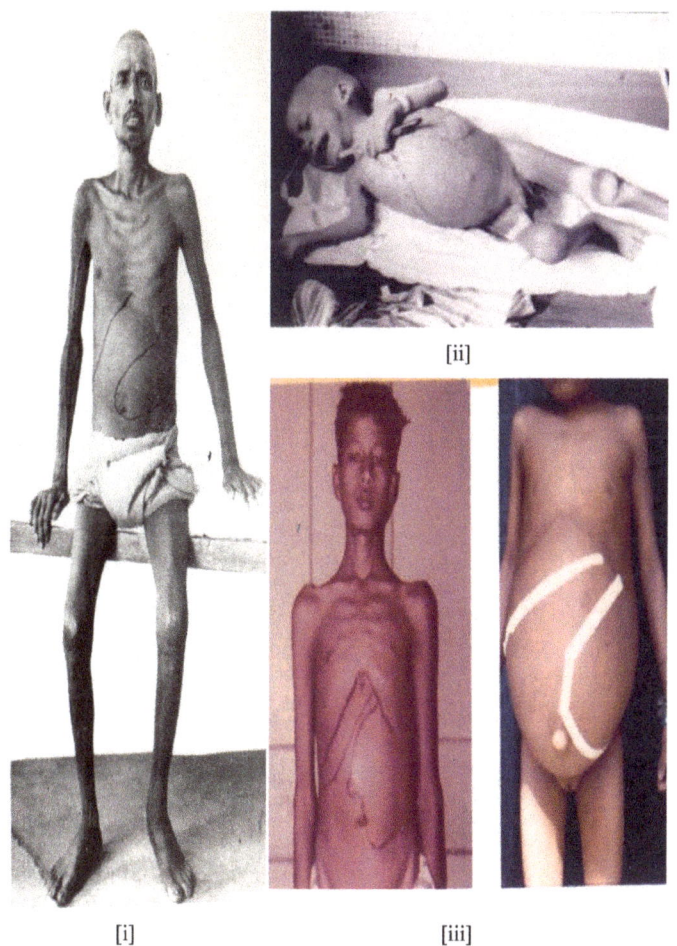

[ii]

[i]   [iii]

FIG.1E (I - III):   Patients with visceral Leishmaniasis

(Courtesy, K.D.Chatterjee, 1975 and Googe web page)

Variation in Visceral Leishmaniasis
Post Kala-azar dermal Leishmaniasis (PKDL)

A skin condition develops in some cases of infection (Fig.1F$_{i,ii}$). It is about 5% to 10% of cases in India and rare in Mediterranean area and South America. About one to two years after inadequate treatment for kala-azar, the condition usually becomes apparent, marked by reddish, depigmented varied size nodules that sometimes become quite disfiguring, found on skin and mainly on face. About 10% of the patients in India develop this and they serve as the reservoir host of infection.

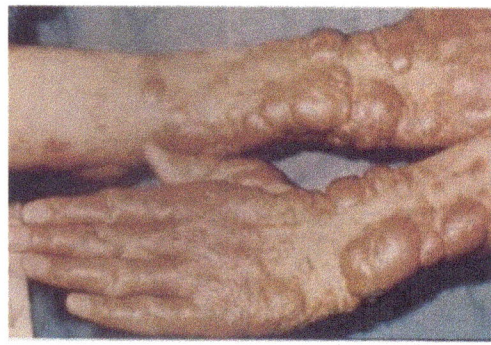

[i]

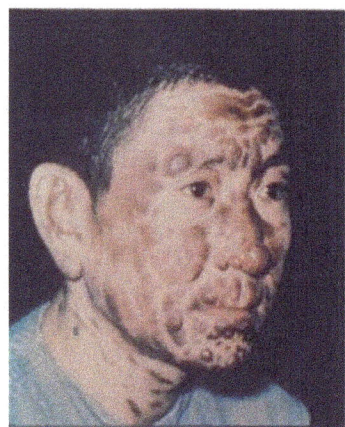

[ii]

FIG. 1 F (I, II)   Skin condition develops following PKDL
(Courtesy, Google web page)

Viscerotropic Leishmaniasis

In viscerotropic Leishmaniasis, an oligo-parasitic condition prevails and it is mainly dermotropic. Visceral infection with *L.tropica* is the causative root of this infection. It was noted among US servicemen in Persian Gulf War during 1990's.

1.1.5.2 Cutaneous Leishmaniasis

The causative agents *L. tropica*, *L. major* phenetic complex along with *L. infantum* phenetic complex ánd *L. braziliensis* (New World) are responsible for cutaneous Leishmaniasis (25).

This disease is found in West Central Africa, Middle East, India, S-Mexico and S-America. They produce cutaneous ulcers variously known as oriental sore, Jericho Boil, Aleppo Boil and Delhi Boil. These ulcers occur in arms, face and lower legs. The lesion may vary in severity according to age and other factors ranging from tiny sores to massive, diffused ulcers. Secondary infection to occur is very common including yaws (a disfiguring disease caused by Spirochete) and myiasis (infection with fly maggots) (10) (Fig.1G$_{i-iii}$).

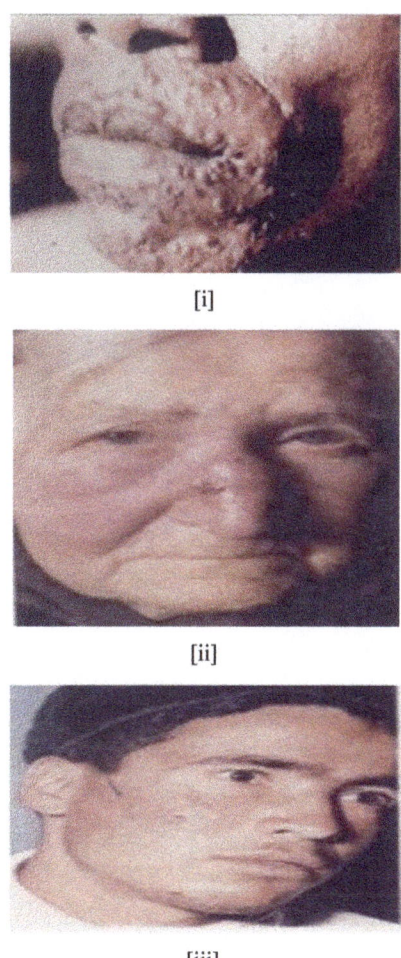

[i]

[ii]

[iii]

FIG.1G (I-III):   Infection with cutaneous Leishmaniasis

(Courtesy: Google web page)

Variations in cutaneous Leishmaniasis
Mucocutaneous Leishmaniasis

The main affected part of the body by Mucocutaneous Leishmaniasis is the nose and mouth. Moreover, lip, gum, palate, buccal cavity, pharynx, larynx, trachea are also affected. It destroys the voice box completely and genitalia may also become infected (10). Granulomatous dermal inflammation (small papulae) develops as a necrotic centre, which enlarges into a massive lesion. The causative agent mainly is *L. brazilliensis brazilliensis* (2). It is found throughout the vast area between central Mexico and Northern Argentina. Morphologically, *L. brazilliensis* cannot be differentiated from *L. tropica, L. mexicana* and *L. donovani*.

Diffuse cutaneous Leishmaniasis

Its causative agents are *L. aethiopica* (Old world) and *L. mexicana* phenetic complex (New world). It develops in the context of Leishmanial specific allergy, which is often misdiagnosed as leprosy or tuberculosis as manifested by non-ulcerative skin lesions. The disease is frequent in Northern and Central America, Mexico, Texas and Trinidad. It infects several thousand persons a year, especially agricultural or forest labourers. This disease usually heads spontaneously in a few months except when the lesions are in the ear (as ear cartilage is poorly vascularized so immune responses are weak) (10).

1.1.6 Pathogenesis

As we are dealing mainly with *L. donovani* parasite, clinically visceral infection of this parasite ranges from asymptomatic to progressive, fully developed kala-azar.

1.1.6.1 Incubation time

In human, the incubation period may be as short as 10 days to as long a year but two to four months on average (10).

1.1.6.2 Symptoms

With low-grade fever, malaise, the disease is followed by profuse wasting, severe anaemia, protrusion of abdomen as a result of enlarged spleen and liver. Fever upto 40°C (104°F) accompanied by chill and vomiting are general symptoms during onset followed by edema of face, breathing problem, bleeding of mucous membranes and diarrhea. The invasion of the secondary pathogen that the body is unable to combat results in immediate death (33, 10). However, a certain proportion of cases in India, recover spontaneously. A skin condition usually becomes apparent in about one to two years of inadequate treatment of kala-azar, called PKDL, marked by depigmented nodules and disfigured facial appearance, reddish in colour (10).

1.1.6.3 Splenic changes

Enlarged, bulky spleen can be observed macroscopically. Spleen can be cut easily, with marked congestion at the site. Tissue becomes friable. Widely dilated vascular spaces and increased reticular cells, densely packed with amastigotes of *L.donovani* are viewable microscopically. Parenchyma devoid of fibrosis with thin and a trophic trabeculae develops. To the detriment of RBC production, spleen may undergo compensatory production of macrophages and other phagocytes (hyperplasia) (34).

1.1.6.4 Hepatic transformation

Liver is congested and enlarged. Increased size in Kupffer's cells with densely filled amastigotes of *L. donovani* and dilated sinusoidal capillaries can be viewed microscopically. Liver cells become devoid of parasites and may undergo atrophy. No increase of fibrous tissue occurs.

1.1.6.5 Change in bone marrow

Bone marrow also undergoes compensatory production of macrophages and other phagocytes, a condition called hyperplasia. Several hinderances in the activities of haematopoietic system of bone marrow occur as a result of infection.

1.1.6.6 Transformation in other organs

As a result of secondary infection, intestinal ulcer occurs. In some areas of China, lymph nodes are infected. Jaundice may develop due to infection of liver.

1.1.7 Immunology

Experiments have shown that experimental animals respond in a different way to visceral parasites though *L. donovani* has not been studied to quite the extent of other species at least in mice in the context of Immunology. Membrane lipophosphoglycans are possessed by *L.donovani* that may inhibit macrophage gene expression. The inhibition is of protein kinase-dependent expression type, such as that involved in macrophage activation by TNF-α and IFN-γ (35). The relationship between host genetic make up and the immunological response to Leishmanial infection has been studied extensively in mice. Susceptibility of mice to *L. donovani* infection is controlled by a single gene Lsh, which is inherited in Mendelian fashion and expressed in Visceral Leishmaniasis (10).

1.1.8 Diagnosis

Leishmanial disease diagnosis is dependent on finding LD bodies in tissues or secretion. Tests based on the following procedures are used:

- Spleen punctures, blood or nasal smears, bone marrow and other tissues are examined for the parasites, and cultures from these organs are attempted.
- Testing for delayed hypersensitivity to *Leishmania* (Montenegro or Leishman test).
- To assay the presence either of non-specific changes in serum proteins or of anti-Leishmanial antibody or of both (4), Serodiagnosis should be done.
- ELISA and indirect fluorescent antibody test (IFA) are also done nowadays as the main limitation of these tests was a cross-reacting positive response to *Trypanosoma cruzi*, which was resolved by improved techniques of antigen purification, specific antigen polymerization and antigen selection by the use of monoclonal antibodies (36). Other diseases like typhoid to paratyphoid, fever, malaria, etc. may have similar symptoms like

kala-azar and each must be eliminated during kala-azar diagnosis. Various laboratory procedures are adopted for kala-azar diagnosis (12) (Table 1B), (Fig. 1H).

TABLE- 1B: Diagnosis of Kala-azar
Laboratory Diagnosis of Kala-azar

Direct Evidence (Demonstration of *L.donovani*)			Indirect Evidences		
Peripheral Blood by thick film method.	Blood culture in N.N.N.	Biopsy material obtained by	Blood count -Leucopenia (progessive)	Serum tests	
Amastigotes form*	Medium. Promastigote form**				
Lymph node puncture	Sternalor iliac crest puncture (Marrow)	Spleen puncture (splenic pulp)	Aldehyde test- positive after 3 months	Antimony test- less reliable	Complement fixation test with W.K.K. antigen

* Amastigote form in a stained smear.
** Promastigote form in culture (N.N.N. medium).

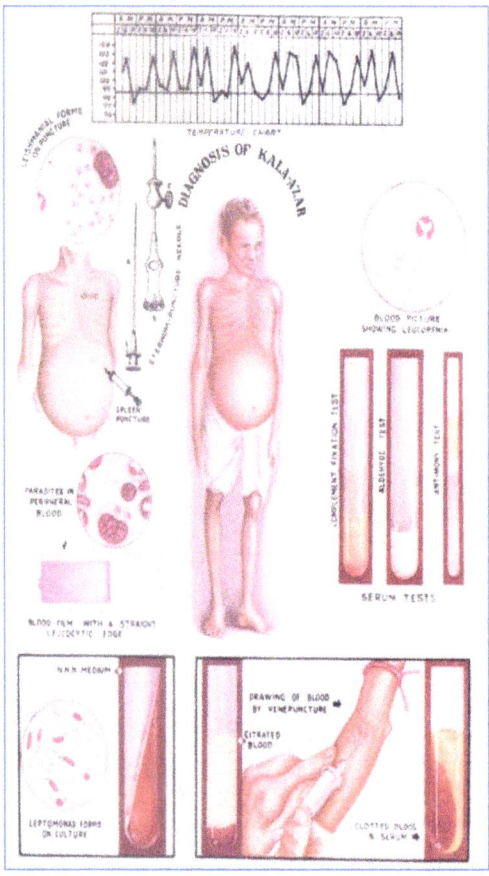

FIG. 1H: Procedures adopted for Kala-azar diagnosis

(Courtesy, K.D.Chatterjee, 1975)

1.1.9 Epidemiology, control and treatment

Biology of sandflies and activities of humans is related to the transmission of visceral Leishmaniasis. Thus, in endemic areas, control of sandflies and reservoir hosts is required. *Phlebotomus* sp. exist most commonly in flat plains at altitudes under 2000 ft. The fly rests in cracks in the parched earth and under rocks which offer protection. The flies are active during certain hours of the day. For humans to be infected, they must be in sandfly areas at these times (10). Although Canine infection is predominant in rest of the world but very rare in India, where it is believed that a fly to human relationship is maintained. Age and sex are two most important factors in the course of infection. Fatal outcome is most frequent in infants and small children (low immunity). Males are more prone to infection than females for more exposure to sandflies, poor nutrition, concomitant infection with other pathogens and stress factors, which predispose the patient to lethal consequences (10). Until now, treatment (Table lC) consists of intravenous or intramuscular injection of various antimonial compounds and good nursing care, although these antimonials are too toxic and sometimes resistant (37). Relapses and PKDL may follow insufficient treatment.

TABLE-1C: Important clinically used anti-Leishmanial drugs

Drug	Syndrome	Dosage regimen
Parenteral		
Pentavalent antimony	VL	20 mg Sb(V)/Kg daily for 28 days
(Intravenous or intramuscular)	CL	20 mg Sb(V)/Kg daily for 20 days
	ML	20 mg Sb(V)/Kg daily for 28 days
Amphotericin B		0.5-1.0 mg/kg on alternate days or
deoxycholate (intravenous)	VL	daily total about 15-20 mg/kg)
	CL	1 mg/kg on alternate days or
	ML	daily (total about 20-40 mg/kg)
		2-5 mg/kg daily (total about 15-21mg/kg)
Lipid formulations of	VL	
Amphotericin B (intravenous)	CL, ML	Not currently recommended
Pentamidine isethionate		4 mg/kg on alternate days or three times/wk
(intravenous or intramuscular)	VL	for about 15-30 doses
	CL	3 mg/kg on alternate days x 4 doses or
		2 mg/kg on alternate days x 7 doses
	ML	2-4 mg/kg on alternate days or three times
		per week for 15 or more doses
Paromomycin sulphate	VL	15-20 mg/kg daily for about 21 days
(intravenous or intramuscular)	CL	Not currently recommended
Recombinant interferon gamma		100 µg/m² daily or on alternate days
subcutaneous or intramuscular)		(adult dose)
Oral		
Ketoconazole	CL	600 mg daily for 28 days (adult dose)

TABLE-1C: *Cont.*

Drug	Syndrome	Dosage regimen
Itraconazole	CL	200 mg twice daily for 28 days (adult dose)
Dapsone	CL	100 mg twice daily for 6 weeks (adult dose)
Paromomycin sulphate ointment	CL	
Intralesional Sb(V)	CL	

1.2 Macrophage: Basic Biology

1.2.1 Origin

One of the prime cells of the mononuclear phagocytic system is the macrophage. This cell system consists of bone marrow monoblasts and promonocytes, blood monocytes and motile and non-motile macrophages of the tissues. Ranges of their distribution vary widely throughout the body exhibiting vast heterogeneity of structure and function (38). Macrophages are active, motile, adherent and highly phagocytic. Moreover, they can be activated by lymphokines. They bear a variety of antigens and receptors on their surfaces and have significant role in immune responses and endocytosis involving receptor-ligand interaction (39).

Precursor Cells

Macrophage's root of origin underlies in the bone marrow stem cells. Resident macrophages and also their precursors, monoblasts, promonocytes, monocytes all reside within the bone marrow. The first progenitor cells of the mononuclear phagocyte system are the monoblasts (38). These are round, 10-12 µm in diameter. From the division of monoblast, promonocytes are obtained, which are 15µm in diameter (38, 40). From precursor promonocytes of the bone marrow, the monocytes are formed.

Monocytes

From the bone marrow the monocytes are released into the blood. In the blood, they are distributed into two pools, namely, circulating and migrating monocytes (41). Migration of blood monocytes to extravascular tissues and to target organs glorifies them to mature as macrophages. About 10-20µm in diameter, with large nucleus, the monocyte has abundant cytoplasm and has a fine granular texture due to the presence of high amount of lysosomal granules. These mononuclear phagocytic cells engulf particles including infectious agents thereby internalising and abolishing them. They are thus strategically placed, where the encounter with such particles will be easier, for example, Synovial A cells line the synovial cavity and Kupffer cells of liver line the sinusoids.

Macrophage

"Professional" phagocytic macrophages are derived from bone marrow cells of the mononuclear phagocytic system. Myeloid progenitor cells in the bone marrow differentiate into promonocytes and then into blood monocytes. Cells from this circulating pool migrate through the blood vessel walls into the various organs and tissue systems to become macrophages (38).

1.2.2 Distribution

Phagocytic macrophages are found in many organs and on the basis of their presence, they are classified as histocytes in connective tissues, Kupffer cells in liver, intraglomerular mesangium of the kidney, alveolar macrophage in the lung, serosal macrophage, brain microglia, spleen sinus macrophage, lymph node sinus macrophage and peritoneal macrophage. Macrophages indigenous to different organs are differed in basic structure and function (42, 38). In response to chemotactic stimuli like complement factors, bacterial products, etc. migration of macrophages can occur.

1.2.3 Properties

Macrophage adheres strongly to glass and plastic surfaces and actively phagocytose the organism or even tumour cells *in vitro*. Adherance and ingestion by macrophage occurs when the cells bind the microorganisms through specialised receptors. The receptors may bind to certain carbohydrates of the microbial cell wall or to lgG and complement with which the microorganism becomes coated.

1.2.4 Isolation and Purification of macrophages

In experimental studies mainly, spleen, peritoneal exudate, bone marrow and lymph node derived macrophages, usually, macrophages are separated from lymphocytes, by adherence to glass or plastic surface or by passing the complex cells suspensions over columns of glass beads or sephadex. From lymphocytes, macrophages can be separated by velocity sedimentation and buoyant density centrifugation. The most reliable technique for separating a macrophage from a lymphocyte is by adherance, although, macrophage cannot be prepared free of lymphocytes absolutely.

Macrophage as a useful model

Macrophage is useful to study membrane organization and function as the functions of these mononuclear phagocyte systems that occur in plasma membrane are all interrelated. Large amount of cells can be obtained from alveolar wash fluid and peritoneal exudates for composition analysis of isolated membranes. Living macrophages can be maintained for greater time period for tissue culture experiments and radioactive tracer techniques. Macrophages contain several surface receptors and thus enable us to study surface topography. During a physiologically significant cell activity, macrophage membrane is sampled for the distribution of surface markers (43) as it is capable of removing a large proportion of the plasma membrane during pinocytosis and phagocytosis.

1.2.5 Classification of macrophages

Resident macrophages

Without the addition of an external inflammatory agent, peritoneal or alveolar macrophages, obtained from animal are called resident/non-stimulated/non-elicited macrophages (44, 45). Macrophages occurring in normal, non-inflamed tissues, in specific sites are also called resident macrophages (38). These cells adhere readily to surfaces over which they move by amoeboid motion. They are active phagocytes and cytodestructive to cells that they ingest.

Elicited macrophages

Introduction of an irritant as thioglycollate broth, protease, peptone, adjuvant, sodium caseinate or mineral oil can result in the formation of elicited macrophages (46). These cells are attracted to a given site because of a particular stimulus. These macrophages have neutral proteases, alterations in content of several ectoenzymes, increased size and high content of acid hydrolases (47-49).

Activated macrophages

Animals immunologically sensitised to specific antigens or following bacterial infection result in the formation of activated macrophages (45). Nonspecifically enhanced activities are displayed by these cells against microorganisms and cells (44). Activated macrophages present antigens to T-cells, destroy tumour cells and facultative or obligate intracellular parasites (47).

Comparison of resident, elicited and activated macrophages

Resident macrophages exhibit low spreading and diminished secretion of plasminogen activator than elicited macrophages. Elicited macrophages, on the other hand, do not release substantial level of toxic forms of oxygen (H_2O_2) and also do not exhibit microbicidal or tumoricidal activity (50, 51). Chemically elicited and immunologically activated macrophages are similar with respect to increase in oxidative burst (52) and decrease in 5' nucleotidase enzyme activity (49). In comparison to elicited macrophages, activated macrophages exhibit low levels of ectoenzyme alkaline phosphodiesterase production, elevated H_2O_2 generation, increased secretion of novel cytolytic protease and binding of tumour cells (53-57).

1.2.6 Activation of macrophages

Activated macrophages are those cells having acquired increased capacity to destroy various pathogens (intra or extra-cellular) and to lyse or inhibit the proliferation of suitable target cells, through enzymatic activation or through stimulation of certain metabolic pathways and enzymatic activities.

1.2.6.1 Mechanism of activation of macrophages

Macrophage activation is a complex phenomenon. Immune response involving stimulation of antigen-specific T-lymphocytes leads to macrophage activation (36, 58, 59). These inturn release a variety of lymphokines (60), displaying activating properties (61). The best known macrophage-activating factors are IFN-γ GMCSF (granulocyte-macrophage colony stimulating factor (62) and TNF-α (63). Activation occurs in stages and requires sequential stimulus, possible stimuli include lymphokines, endotoxins, various mediators and regulators of inflammation (63). A variety of stimuli can induce the morphological, functional and biochemical changes (36, 64-66). Macrophages can also become activated by interaction with antigen-antibody complexes (67-69), double stranded RNA (70, 71), endotoxin (72, 73) and complement component pathway (74, 75). Growth hormones and other structurally and functionally related molecules are also found to activate macrophages (76, 77). Different effector functions may be expressed at each stage and there are characteristic changes in macrophage appearance and physiology.

1.2.6.2 Heterogeneity

Activated macrophages show enhanced ability to kill some micro-organisms, but not others. The reasons for this complexity are:

- Activated macrophages can express numerous different effector functions.
- Macrophage series is very heterogeneous; cells taken from different sites differ in relevant characteristics (38, 42).
- The functions activated may depend not only on the macrophage but also on the precise "blend" of lymphokines and inflammatory stimuli to which it is exposed.

1.2.7 Macrophage features

1.2.7.1 Morphology

In light microscopic view, macrophages can be described as large, irregular cells with oval or kidney-shaped nucleus (38). Cytoplasm is abundant of fine and large granules. Near the cell periphery, the cytoplasmic vacuoles are found, reflecting active phagocytosis.

In phase contrast microscope, highly ruffled cell membranes with large cells which spread on glass surfaces with the cell organelles concentrated within the central region (78) are observed.

Electron microscopic view reveals a cytoplasm with scattered strands of RER, variable number of vesicle and vacuoles, a well-characterised golgi complex, large mitochondria and electron dense membrane bound lysosomes which can be seen fusing with phagosomes to form secondary lysosomes. Microfilaments and microtubules are very prominent in macrophages (33).

1.2.7.2 Macrophage membrane and its composition

Characterization of macrophage membrane is important in understanding the molecular mechanism associated with the biological events. Phagocytosis, pinocytosis, antigen binding, cell recognition, etc. are some of the biological events in which macrophages participate.

Membrane morphology

Macrophages have a plasma membrane, trilammelar in structure having unaccountable vesicles close to the membrane (79). The cell coat is 8-16 nm thick. Extremely ruffled and folded plasma membrane and multiple pseudopodia with cup or funnel-like shapes can be scanned during phagocytosis (80, 81).

Membrane composition

Macrophage membrane contains 46% protein, 41% lipid, 8% carbohydrate and 3% RNA. The membrane-associated processes like cell locomotion, spreading, adherance, endocytosis and membrane organization are all dependent on the cytoskeletal microtubule-microfilament system. The cytoskeletal matrix consists of two regions - a random oriented matrix and a zone of oriented bundles of microfilaments and microtubules (82).

Membrane organization

Macrophage activation by pathogenic strains of parasites can alter the receptor expression (57, 83, 84). A change in membrane microviscosity can modulate the receptor expression of cells in general (85). Pervasive use of membranes is one of the most important features of cellular organization. Plasma membrane not only binds the cell at their surface but also provides space for performing specific cellular functions. The knowledge of structural organization of a membrane is important to understand its functional activities. In 1972, Singer & Nicolson proposed a 'fluid mosaic model' of the membrane (Fig.1L), (131). The phospholipids of membranes are arranged in a bilayer to form a fluid, liquid crystalline matrix or core.

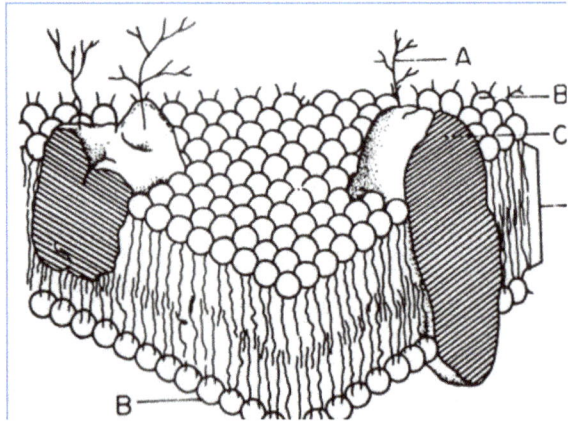

FIG. 1L: Fluid mosaic model; A-sugar residue; B-polar phospholipid head group; C- intrinsic membrane proteins; D-hydrophobic fatty acyl chains

Membrane fluidity or membrane microviscosity

Exhibition of varying degrees of mobility (or fluidity) is expressed by membrane components. Membrane exhibits varying degrees of mobility (or fluidity) under normal temperature. Not only the degree of unstaturation of the hydrocarbon chains, the fluidity of a given lipid, also varies with the length of it. From the fluidity of the lipid matrix, the mobility of the integral proteins arises in the membrane. In mammalian membrane, cholesterol is present for maintenance of membrane fluidity. During severe alterations in mobility of phospholipid acyl chains, cholesterol acts as buffer (86, 87).

Measurement of membrane fluidity or membrane microviscosity

All molecules having a set of energy level S1, S2, etc., within each of which different vibrational levels remain, provides further subdivision. Most molecules are in the lowest vibrational level of the ground electronic state at RTM. The molecule is excited to the excited singlet state S_1 or to a higher state, after absorption of Energy "E".

By a number of pathways they can return to the ground state. Direct demotion to an intermediate vibrational state of S_0 can occur with emission of energy and this process is known as fluorescence. Immediate environment polarity of a molecule affects the electronic and vibrational energy levels. The polarity of the environment and viscosity is very sensitive for the fluorescent probes. The mobility of the fluorescent probe can also be assessed and used to report on the viscosity of its immediate environment. Excitation of the probe with a plane-polarized light will lead to the emission of light polarized in the same plane or perpendicular to the plane of polarization of the excitation beam (86, 88, 89). The total fluorescence intensity F is calculated as $F = I_{\parallel} + 2\, l_{\perp}$, where $l_{\parallel}$ and $I_{\perp}$ are the fluorescence intensities detected through a polarizer oriented parallel and perpendicular to the direction of polarization of the excited beam. The degree of fluorescence polarization P_1 reflects the mobility of the fluorophores. P is expressed as fluorescence anisotropy, r. As the parameter 'P' reflects the mobility of the fluorophore it can be used to obtain a value for the microviscosity of the environment. One form of Perrin's Equation on which the determinations of fluorescence polarization are based is

$$r_0 / r = 1 + 3\,\tau\, / \rho$$

where, τ is the life time of the excited state of the fluorophore and ρ is the rotational relaxation time. The term r_0 is the maximal limiting anisotrophy which for DPH (diphenyl hexatrene) is 0.362 (87, 90).

Membrane Antigens

On the surface of macrophages, several surface antigens as Ia (91, 92), MHC antigen and Mac-1 (93) are present. In response to exogenous signals, expression of Ia antigen is regulated and is associated with antigen presentation to lymphocytes (91, 92).

1.2.8 Macrophage cell markers/Macrophage cell receptors

Interaction of the immune system with the microbial world involves molecules known as microbial pattern recognition receptors present in macrophages (94). The interaction of *Leishmania* parasites with macrophage is known to be receptor-mediated (95) and that involves surface membrane proteins (96). Receptor interactions are important determinants of the infectivity and survival of *Leishmania* parasites in the vertebrate (97). Macrophage activities like growth, differentiation, activation, recognition, endocytosis, migration and secretion are controlled by a large number of cell surface markers. They include Integrin receptors, complement receptors, MFR, AGE receptor, LFA-l, HLA-D, etc., involving receptor ligand interaction. Though by the receptors extracellular signals are received and transduced across the cell membrane, regulation of microbicidal, tumoricidal activities and macrophage activation were studied by various researchers by ligating specific receptors (98, 99). The various receptors present on phagocytes including macrophage surface are summarized in Table 1D, 1E.

TABLE 1D: Adhesion and Phagocytosis Receptors on Macrophages

Receptors	Ligands
Integrins	
CR3 P150/95 LFA- 1 Fibronectin / VLA— 5 VLA-2 Laminin	C3bi, gp63,fibrinogen,LPS, LPG C3bi, LPS, LPG ICAM-1, LPS Fibronectin Collagen Laminin
Complement receptors	
CR1 Fc Fc RI Fc RII	C3b, C3bi Monomeric IgG Complexed IgG
Carbohydrate receptors	
Mannosyl/ fucosyl	Glycoconjugates with terminal D-Mannose, L-fucose, N-acetyl-D-glucosamine or D-glucose
Advanced gycosylated end product (AGE)	Glucosylated moieties

TABLE 1E: Surface Receptors of monocytes and macrophages

Category	Receptors
Cytokine receptor	MIF, MAF, IL-I, IL-2, IL-3, IL-4, IFN-α, IFN-β, IFN-γ, GMCSF, CSF-1
Receptors for peptides and small molecules	N-formylated peptides, 1,2,5 Dihydroxy Vitamin D3, Enkephalins, Substance-P, Arg-Vasopressin.
Hormone Receptors, Transferrin and lactoferrin receptors	Insulin, Glucocorticoids, Angiotensin

Lipoprotein lipid receptors	Anionic low density lipoproteins, PGE-2 Apolipoprotein B and E.
Receptors for coagulants and anticoagulants	Fibrinogen/Fibrin, Coagulation factor VII α-1 antithrombin, Heparin
Fibronectin receptors Laminin receptors Mannosyl fucosyl, galactosyl residue, AGE receptor α-2 -Macroglobulin-proteinase complex receptors Others	Cholinergic agonist, α-and β-2 Adrenergic agonist

1.2.8.1 Mannosyl Fucosyl Receptor (MFR Receptor or MR Receptor)

MFR is one of the most well characterised receptors (100) expressed on macrophages (101,164,173,175,177). The receptor mediates uptake of intracellular parasites *L. donovani* (102), *T. cruzi* (103) by macrophages. For the complement independent clearance of pathogenic organisms that have polymannose structures on their membranes (eg. *Candida albicans*), macrophage plays a role in the immune system (104). Mannose fucose receptors are important in promastigotes binding and respiratory burst activity (105). Uptake and degradation of high mannose type oligosaccharides containing glycoproteins (as lysosomal enzymes) are mediated by receptor (106). Functional state of macrophage is regulated and correlates with the expression of receptor. This MFR is not expressed by monocytes and higher levels of these receptors are expressed by resting macrophage than activated macrophage (57,107,108,109). These receptors recognise glycoproteins having terminal mannose, N-acetyl glucosamine or fucose as terminal residues of various lysosomal glycosidases. The surface and cell wall of infectious agents are decorated by various patterns of carbohydrates which are recognised by mannose receptor that mediates the endocytosis of infectious agent. This receptor is trypsin sensitive and requires Ca^{2+} for binding. 180 kDa transmembrane protein MFR, has 5 domains (110): the amino terminal cysteine rich region, a domain containing fibronectin type II repeat, a series of eight tandem lectin like carbohydrate recognition domains (CRDS), a transmembrane domain and a cytoplasmic domain (Fig. 1 J). A first line of host defense and antigen presentation of lipophosphoglycan antigens (111), is performed by MR. When engaged by microorganisms or particles, MR induces signal transduction that triggers a variety of responses including secretion of lysosomal enzymes (112) and production of O_2^- (113), cytokines (114, 115). A more passive role in phagocytosis of pathogens is played by MR.

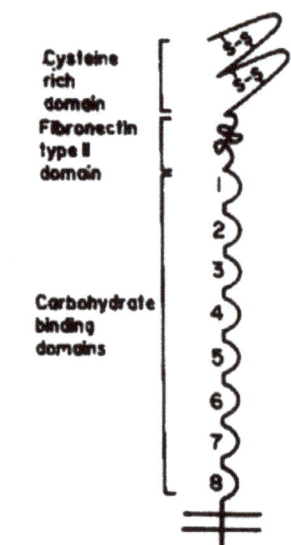

FIG. 1J: Schematic representation of Mannose receptor

1.2.8.2 Integrin receptors

The integrins are a large family of α/β heterodimeric transmembrane receptors, expressed by a variety of cell types (116). In cultured mammalian cells, β_1 integrins and other cytoskeletal proteins such as vinculin, talin, actin and paxillin are localized at sites of cellular adhesion to the extracellular matrix (ECM) (focal adhesions). A single domain of invasin corresponding to the 192 carboxyterminal residues is sufficient to mediate attachment and entry (117,118). This small region of invasin and fibronectin binds to mutually exclusive site on the integrin receptor $\alpha_5\beta_1$ (119), Fig.1K. Integrins are thought to link extracellular binding events functionally to the cytoskeleton by transduction of signals into the eukaryotic cell (116). Tyrosine phosphorylation plays a key role in signal transduction through integrins (119). Integrin receptor CR3 binds to C3bi, Glycoprotein (gp63), lipophosphoglycan (LPG) (120,121) of the parasite. Parasites are thought to interact with integrins either directly or by absorption of integrin ligands such as complement component C3bi to their surfaces (119). Among the integrins, CR3, P150/95, LFA-I, VLA- 2, Laminin are important ones that are involved in phagocytosis and adhesion (120, 121, 166-169, 171, 172, 392).

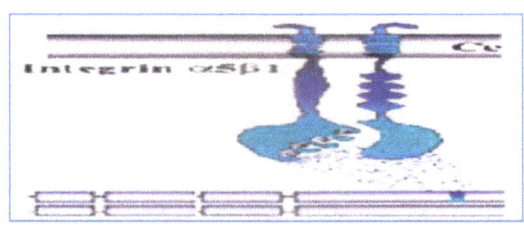

[i]

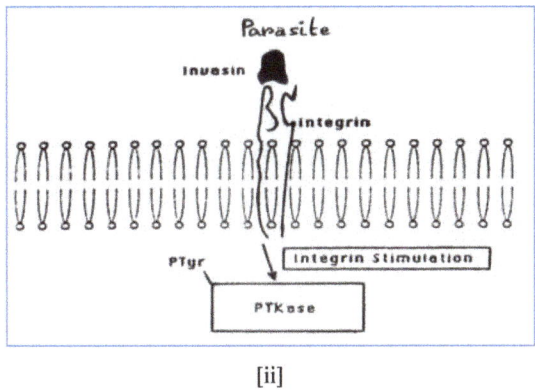

[ii]

FIG. 1K: (i) shows the structure of integrin receptor (ii) shows a model for parasite-host cell interaction. Parasite interacted with invasin to a host cell β integrin receptor. Parasite entry is hypothesized to be stimulated by invasion-integrin complex, which tiggers activation of a PTKase and leads to tyrosine phosphorylation (PTyr) of a PTKase. Activation of this PTKase is proposed to initiate intimate parasite attachment and entry by facilitating the transduction of signals to the host-cell interaction.

1.2.8.3 Complement receptors

Opsonization of promastigotes with the third component of complement promotes their adhesion to macrophage complement receptor, thus complement receptors are the cleavage products of the third component of complement, C3b, C3bi (47). CR1 recognises C3b and CR3 recognises C3bi (38). Macrophages bind to C3-coated particles, though the expression of CR3 receptors is lost in those cells that are elicited with inflammatory stimuli (123). CRI (CD35) and Mac-1 (CR3, CD18, 11b), bind preferentially to C3b and ic3b respectively. The adhesion of parasites to CR1 is very transient because of the factor 1 co-factor activity of CR1, which facilitates the cleavage activity of C3b to ic3b and gp63 can cleave C3b to ic3b. Mac-1 is the primary complement receptor that firmly adheres to host complement receptor during phagocytosis (124). CR1 mediates the initial complement dependent adhesion of parasites to macrophages (124). Macrophage receptor C3bi (CR3) plays a major role in phagocytosis of parasites even in absence of serum (125). Less respiratory burst is provoked by CR1 receptor and thus thought to be better for internalisation and survival of parasites (126, 127). Evasion of the complement cascade by *Leishmania* is an integral part of the parasite's life cycle. The alternative pathway of complement is activated by most species of *Leishmania* (128, 129).

Inflammatory macrophage binds and phagocytoses C3bi-coated particles via C3b receptors while resident macrophage binds but cannot ingest these particles via these receptors.

Uptake of zymosan and *L. donovani* in macrophage is mediated via MFR and CR3. Complement dependent opsonisation not only improves their adhesion to macrophage but also enhances their intracellular survival (11).

1.2.8.4 IFN-γ Receptor

Antiviral, antiproliferative and immunoregulatory effects are some of the diverse functional consequences of IFN-γ in various cell types (130). Activation of a protein kinase and induction of rise in intracellular levels of Ca^{2+} are the most important biochemical changes involved. IFN-γ initiates a very complex type of signalling events. Both Murine and human IFN-γ bind in a species-specific manner to their respective receptors and induce biological functions or responses.

1.3 Host parasite interaction: Attachment and Internalisation

Intracellular parasitism of host macrophage is the pathologic hallmark of Leishmaniasis (132). A dual role is played by the macrophage in Leishmaniasis by playing both as host as well as immunoregulator and effector cell of the parasite. This host-parasite interaction determines the results of all microbial infection (122, 133-138). Parasites deal with both the intracellular as well as extracellular microenvironments of the host. Plasma membrane of macrophage is involved in a crucial role in antimicrobial activities (139). Microorganisms are attached to the surface receptors of macrophages and are phagocytosed into the phagosome. Fusion of phagosome and lysosome exposes parasites to microbicidal factors. Activated macrophage apart from inactivated one elicits protective immune responses (150). To kill intracellular parasite, parasite-(antigen) specific lymphocytes and their secretory products activate macrophages. The two important cytokines secreted by the lymphocytes are IFN-γ and TNF-α, which activate macrophages to generate reactive oxygen metabolites eg, O_2^-, OH^-, $^1O_2$, H_2O_2 (140-144) and reactive nitrogen metabolites as - nitric oxide (NO) via L-arginine catabolism in macrophages (146,148,149,153). For antiparasitic activity, both ROl and RNI are important (145-149,151,152). The generation of cytokines viz TNF-α and IFN-γ (TH-1 response) and IL-4, lL-10 (TH-2 response) are important for destruction and survival of the parasite inside the host respectively (144,154-159). Leishmania once internalised evades microbicidal machinery of host and safely survives inside the phagolysosomal compartment of the host macrophage.

Macrophage-*Leishmania* interactions can be sequentially interpreted as follows:

1.3.1 Chemotaxis

1.3.2 Recognition of *Leishmania* on the macrophage surface via receptor ligand binding and their subsequent attachment

1.3.3 Entry of *Leishmania* by a process called receptor-mediated endocytosis

1.3.4 Macrophage membrane signalling

1.3.5 Triggering of microbicidal responses of macrophages

1.3.1 Chemotaxis

Directed movement of macrophages along a concentration gradient of a chemical factor is described as chemotaxis (134). Specific receptors on cell surface are bound by chemo-attractant and initiate the leukocyte response. Soluble bacterial factors C5a, C5, C6, C7, tuftsin, IFN-γ, N-formylated peptides, etc. are the macrophage chemotaxins. These chemotaxins are expressed as the surface receptors by macrophages along with their engagement in respiratory burst activation and lysosomal enzyme degranulation (47, 160). Bray, 1983 (388) has demonstrated a number of substances chemotactic for *Leishmania* promastigotes.

1.3.2 Recognition of parasite ligand by host receptor and their subsequent attachment

1.3.2.1 Receptor-ligand interaction

Receptor interactions are important determinant of the attachment, entry, infectivity and survival of *Leishmania* parasites in the vertebrate (162, 139, 170). *Leishmania* gets entry within macrophage via receptor-mediated endocytosis for which macrophage surface receptors are exploited for binding with parasite surface ligands (139, 162). The macrophage receptors (Table 1D, 1E) are involved in binding and internalisation of wide range of ligands among which integrins (120, 121, 166-169, 171, 172), complement receptor (CR1/CR3) (161, 163-165), MFR (164, 173, 175, 177, 102), advanced glycosylated end product receptor (AGE) (176) are most important and involved in phagocytosis and adhesion (179). Binding of *Leishmania* to macrophage occurs either independently or in presence of serum opsonins (Fig.1L).

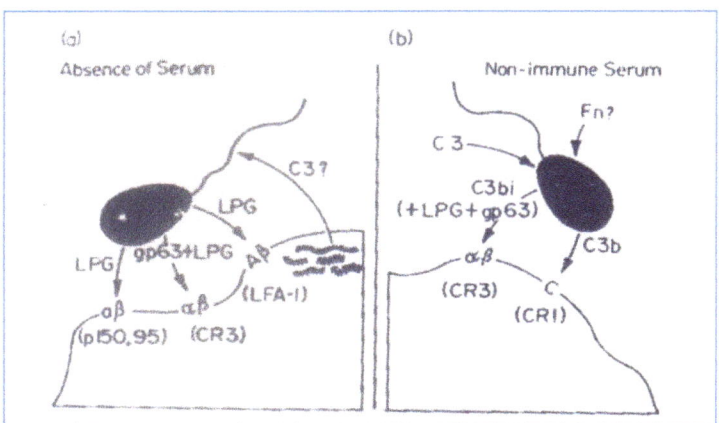

FIG 1L: Binding of Leishmania to macrophages a) in absence of serum; b) In presence of serum opsonins

Binding of *Leishmania* to macrophage, independent of serum

Leishmania attachment with macrophage can occur via CR3, the receptor for C3bi, a fragment of the third component of complement. Macrophage produces C3, which might opsonize *Leishmania* locally under serum-free conditions (162, 164). Non-infected stages of *Leishmania* do not require serum for attachment (126). MFR (102, 178) and fibronectin receptors (FnR) are also utilised in the binding of *Leishmania* to macrophage.

Binding of *Leishmania* to macrophage, dependent on serum

This binding is mediated via adsorption of opsonins (eg., complement and antibodies) by promastigotes and subsequent binding of promastigotes to Fc and CR1 receptors on macrophage. CR1 is the major binding molecule for complement-opsonized metacyclic promastigotes (179). Infected stages of *Leishmania* depend on serum opsonization for entry (126).

1.3.2.2 *Leishmania* surface molecules involved in binding to macrophage

A glycolipid moiety - Lipophosphoglycan (LPG), a ligand found on the surface (180-182, 393) and a glycoprotein (gp63) (183-185, 389) are important players for promoting binding to macrophage and parasite survival in mammalian hosts. Glycoprotein, gp63 binds to CR3 and LPG binds to CR3, P150, 95 receptors of the integrin family (122). LPG actively influences macrophages and mediates promastigotes attachment at an early stage of phagocytosis to generate phagosome with poor fusogenic properties (186). LPG includes an inositol phosphate-linked lipid anchor and glycan core; both are conserved among *Leishmania* species. This molecule is richly glycosylated, especially in the infectious metabolic forms and therefore, LPG has the potential to serve as the ligand for a number of lectin receptors on macrophage (as by MFR) (11). LPG selectively impairs signal transduction in macrophage (188). The *Leishmania* surface protein gp63 has been identified as a parasite virulence factor (133,189). Both LPG and gp63 can fix complement and because of their property they have shown to associate with Mac-1 (the primary complement receptor). They also exhibit a low level of direct binding to macrophages in the absence of serum. Thus, in this way they establish their potential roles as mediators of parasites adhesion to macrophage (11). *Leishmania* parasites have adapted not only to survive, but also to proliferate for the glycoconjugates on its surface (187).

1.3.2.3 Attachment of *Leishmania* leads to active entry into macrophages

Parasitic protozoa enter into phagocytic cells by so called "Zipper hypothesis" (190-192). A "modified zipper" mechanism was formulated by Aikawa and coworkers (193). Microfilament-based capping reaction may actually play a basic role in the attachment and entry of parasite, *Leishmania* into host cells (194-196) (Fig.1M).

The parasite attachment followed by entry involves sequential and circumferential interaction of receptors on the phagocyte with ligands on the surface of the parasite (199). This process requires the attachment of the parasite to the macrophage (197). Random attachment of the flagellated promastigotes to mononuclear phagocytes initiates their uptake via circumferential pseudopods (198). This process leads to the polymerisation of actin at the site of ingestion and the internalisation of the particle via an actin-based mechanism (199). Actin is a 42-kDa protein which polymerises into filaments (F-actin), is one of the major constituents of the cytoskeleton (200). Actin and myosin microfilaments interact in the region of receptor-ligand contact (138). Phagosome maturation requires the coordinated interaction of the actin and tubulin-based cytoskeleton (199). The uptake of amastigotes by macrophages involves the co-localization of f-actin, paxillin, talin to phagocytic cups that are formed around amastigotes during internalisation (201).

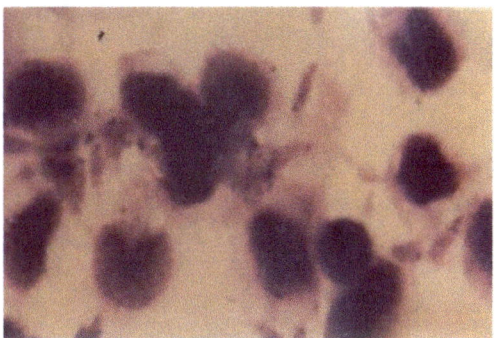

FIG. 1M: Leishmania attached to macrophage

1.3.3 Entry of *Leishmania* into macrophages

1.3.3.1 Receptor-mediated endocytosis

Accumulation of Clathrin-coated pits of the plasma membrane which pinches off continuously to form coated vesicles in the cytosol leads to internalisation of the receptor-ligand complexes (202). Clathrin coat is thus lost and receptor-ligand complexes are delivered to uncoated vesicles called early endosomes (203). Here many ligands dissociate due to a slightly acidic pH and free receptors are returned to the cell surface in recycling vesicles. The ligands are then transported to late endosome (204). Ligands are finally delivered into lysosomes having high acidic pH and high concentration of hydrolytic enzymes as in case of LDL receptors (205). The process is well-demonstrated in parasite binding to macrophage receptors (164).

1.3.3.2 Receptor recycling

Receptor binding to a ligand gets internalised and then delivered to endosomes and efficiently recycled back to plasma membrane (202). LDL receptor and transferrin receptor which are rapidly recycled, discharge their ligands at mildly acidic pH and are then transported back to the plasma membrane. Individual receptors may be reused several times via membrane recycling (206).

1.3.3.3   Modulation of receptors

After receptor-mediated endocytosis, modulation of receptors can take place. Most of the internalised cell surface receptors recycle back to the cell surface (207). But each time a receptor is internalised, there is a probability of the receptor being degraded in the lysosome (217). A receptor protein with a defective coated pit binding site can also lead to down regulation of receptors (208). Macrophage receptors are involved in binding of *Leishmania donovani* promastigotes. Mannose and glucose are specifically involved in binding process.

Receptor expression is increased by treatment with dexamethasone (209,178), Vitamin-D (210), whereas swainsonine (211), IFN-γ (108) and H_2O_2 (212,178) decreases expression. This receptor may participate in a variety of functions involving both up and down regulation of expression. H_2O_2, glucose/glucose oxidants, a prominent constituent of inflammatory milieu are able to down regulate the attachment and internalisation of parasite promastigotes to macrophages (178). The decrease or increase in the uptake is probably due to decrease or increase in the binding of promastigotes (95).

1.3.3.4   Formation of parasitophorous vacuole (PV) and phagolysosome

Intracellular *Leishmania* is surrounded by various types of vacuoles depending on the infecting species and developmental stages of the parasite (213). In *L.donovani* both close fitting vacuole and large vacuole are found (214). *L.donovani* amastigote resides in the parasitophorous vacuole (PV) which is the membrane bound compartment of macrophage (16, 215).

After entering inside the host macrophage by phagocytosis (208, 216), *Leishmania* parasite resides in a phagosome (214, 218), and fuses with the host's secondary lysosome forming phagolysosome (219). Amastigotes of *Leishmania* proliferate in phagolysosomes of mammalian macrophages.

1.3.3.5   Promastigote to amastigote differentiation

Prior to multiplication of the amastigotes in macrophage, intracellular conversion of promastigotes to amastigotes occurs. Depending on the temperature and other factors this differentiation takes place (2), accompanied by antigenic changes (220, 221) (Fig.1 N).

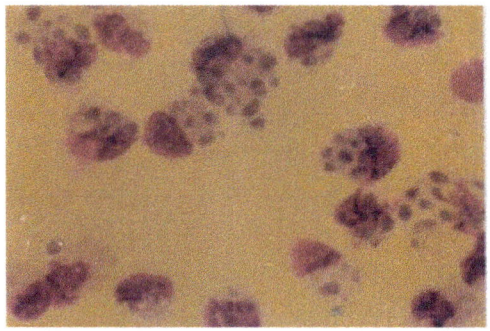

FIG. 1N: Transformation of Leishmania donovani promastigotes to amastigotes inside host macrophages

1.3.4 Macrophage membrane signaling

Extracellular agonists as hormones, growth factors, and adhesion ligands bind and activate receptors in or on target cells. This initiates intracellular events, as the stimulation of intracellular second messengers and thereby activation of signal transduction pathway. Elaborate sets of intracellular signalling proteins form the relay systems. More complex signal transduction involves the coupling of ligand receptor interactions to many intracellular events (208, 222). These intracellular events involve activation of enzyme kinases. These eventually lead to phosphorylation of many proteins. These proteins in turn generally cause the phosphorylation of down stream proteins as part of a phosphorylation cascade. These phosphorylation cascades occur mainly by serine-threonine kinases and tyrosine kinases. The mechanism of signal transduction is shown in Fig. 1.O. Protein phosphorylation changes enzyme activities and protein conformations. The eventual outcome is an alteration in cellular activity. Thus, immediate execution of various complex functions (eg. destruction of microbes) can be stimulated by signals, which can alter the potential of mononuclear phagocytes in order to enhance or diminish their functions. By extracellular signals, macrophage functions are regulated. During interaction of various microorganisms with macrophages or other host cells activate signalling molecules (119,293-295,385) that helps in internalisation of the pathogens. However not much work has been reported in details during *Leishmania* — macrophage interaction, though significant work has been done after internalisation (231, 237-239).

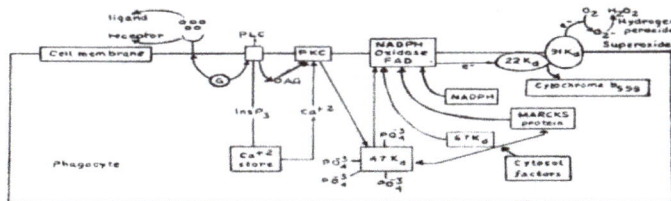

FIG. 1. O: Schematic pathway of PKC-mediated signal transduction.
Signalling of PKC requires: (i) activation of phospholipase C (PLC) and phospholipase D (PLD) after binding of ligand to specific receptor. The signals mediated by a trimeric G protein. (ii) Diacyl glycerol (DAG) and Inositol 4, 5 - triphosphate are generated from breakdown of phosphatidylionositol-4,5-bis phosphate. (iii) binding of IP3 or InsP3 to Ca+2 stores induces the release of Ca+2 to the cytosol. (iv) Ca+2 and DAG activate protein kinase C (PKC) activation of PKC catalyzes the phosphorylation of specific cytosolic proteins (Oxidase factors) including MARCKS (myristic acid rich protein kinase C substrate) which then translocated to the plasma membrane and interact with cytochrome b components of the oxidase and this in turn activates NADPH-oxidase. The functional end points of this signal transduction cascade are superoxide generation.

What are protein kinases?

The largest known protein family is made up of protein kinases. These enzymes use the gamma phosphate of ATP (or GTP) to generate phosphate monoesters i.e., transfer a phosphate group from a phosphate donor (generally, γ phosphate of ATP) onto an acceptor amino acid in a substrate protein (223), utilizing protein alcohol groups (on serine, threonine), protein phenolic groups (on tyrosine) as phosphate group acceptors. They are related by virtue of their homologous "Kinase domains"/"catalytic domains" which consist of ~250-300 amino acid residues (223-225). Several kinases are there among which PTKs and PKCs play key roles in macrophage-parasite interaction.

Protein Tyrosine Kinases (PTKs)

Phosphotransferases with a protein phenolic group as acceptor are called protein-tyrosine kinases (223). There are numerous intracellular PTKs that are responsible for phosphorylating a variety of intracellular proteins on tyrosine residues following activation of cellular growth and proliferation signals. Many families of PTKs, Src-protein, Janus kinase (JaK) have been recognised so far (208). Different families of protein tyrosine kinases mediate a localised rise in tyrosine phosphorylation following receptor ligation (226, 227). PTK-mediated signal transduction involves clustering of integrin receptors (246). Protein tyrosine phosphorylation and dephosphorylation controls various functions of host pathogen interaction by the sequential actions of PTKs and phosphatases (247). Phoshatases antagonise PTK activity (230). Phosphatases are known to play roles in cell adhesion, internalisation and killing of pathogens (248). Alteration of PTK-dependent signalling events are directly responsible for *Leishmania*-induced macrophage dysfunctions (228), *Leishmania* infection blocks tyrosine kinase phosphorylation with impairment of NO production (229). Invasions of virulent or avirulent *L. donovani* promastigotes initiate a host cell PTK-dependent response which signals for actin polymerisation and facilitates the phagocytosis (230). It has been reported that the involvement of protein tyrosine kinases activity in the *Leishmania* attachment, invasion and survival within macrophages, as well as promastigote ability to trigger tyrosine phosphorylation, which could contribute to Leishmanicidal activity (231). Although there are works on PTK, after established infection nothing is known during early phases of interaction i.e., during parasite attachment and entry into macrophages. Fig.1P shows PTK-mediated signal transduction.

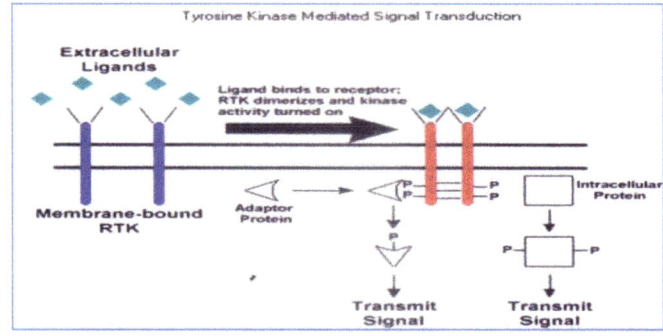

FIG 1P: Mechanism of Protein Tyrosine Kinase-mediated signal transduction

(Courtesy, Google web page)

Protein Kinase C (PKC)

The Ca^{2+} phospholipid-dependent protein kinases (Protein kinase C: PKC) is a protein serine threonine kinase involved in the regulation of many cellular processes including cellular growth, differentiation, tumor promotion (232). The primary structure of PKC has two functional domains, a catalytic domain and a regulatory domain (232). The carboxyl terminal region is the catalytic domain and the amino-terminal region containing cysteine-rich repeats is the regulatory domain having phospholipid and Diacylglycerol (DAG)/Phorbolester binding region. It is known that there are at least ten proteins of the PKC family. Each of these enzymes exhibits specific patterns of tissue expression and activation by lipid and calcium. PKCs are involved in the signal transduction pathway initiated by certain hormones, growth factors and neurotransmitters. The phosphorylation of various proteins by PKC in different cell systems includes phagocytes, which in turn activates NADPH oxidase (234). PKC-mediated signal transduction cascade leads to the generation of superoxide (O_2^-) in phagocytic cells as the functional end-points of the mechanism (235). The mechanism of PKC-mediated signal transduction is shown in Fig. 1Q. PKC translocations and alterations can have global effects on the phagocytic process (238), possibly by influencing events at the cellular cytoskeleton involved in parasite uptake and membrane trafficking. PKC has a regulatory role for cell adhesion and spreading (236). In case of *L. donovani* infection, PKC, the key enzyme for the generation of reactive oxygen intermediates (ROl), is impaired (237-239). There are works on PKC after established infection with the parasite but nothing much is reported during early phase of interaction (attachment of the parasite with the host).

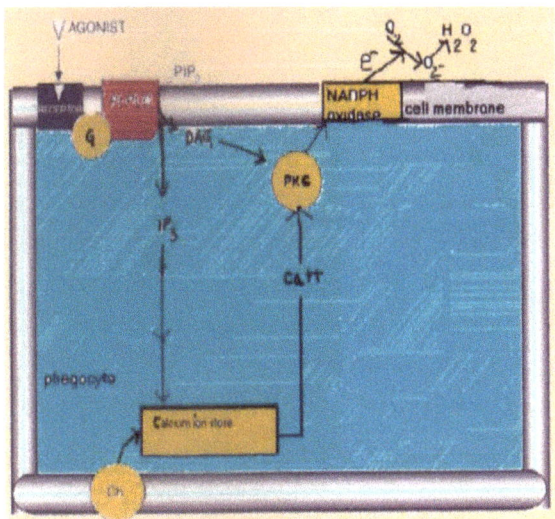

FIG. 1Q: PKC mediated signalling cascade

Signalling of PKC requires: (i) activation of phospholipase C (PLC) and phospholipase D (PLD) after binding of ligand to specific receptor. The signals mediated by a trimeric G protein, (ii) Diacyl glycerol (DAG) and Inositol 4,5 — triphosphate are generated from breakdown of phosphatidylionositol-4,bis phosphate, (iii) binding of IP3 or InsP3 to Ca+2 stores induces the release of Ca+2 to the cytosol, (iv) Ca+2 and DAG activate protein kinase C (PKC) activation of PKC catalyzes the phosphorylation of specific cytosolic proteins (Oxidase factors).

PKC substrates such as MARCKS, MRP, Mac-MARCKS also play role in Leishmanial infection. The roles of these proteins are not clear during early phases of interaction.

The myristoylated alanine-rich C kinase substrate (MARCKS), Macrophage enriched myristoylated alanine rich protein kinase C substrate (Mac-MARCKS) and Macrophage related proteins (MRP) are members of a family of major PKC substrates found in a variety of cells including macrophages (11, 240, 242-245). MARCKS has been proposed to regulate the plasticity of the actin cytoskeleton at its site of attachment to membranes and involves in mobility, adhesion and phagocytosis (241). As MARCKS is a calmodulin and actin binding protein, activation of PKC leads to inhibition of this actin crosslinking activity (245). Thus, the cycle of membrane attachment/detachment represents a mechanism through which PKC might reversibly regulate actin membrane interaction. PKC transduces receptor-mediated signals by phosphorylating membrane bound substrates. PKC-dependent phosphorylation displaces MARCKS from the membrane and that its subsequent dephosphorylation is accompanied by its reassociation with the membrane. Thus, myristoylation of MARCKS is required for effective binding to the plasma membrane where it co-localizes with PKC (242,245). Mac-MARCKS, required for releasing the cytoskeletal constraint on integrin molecules during PKC mediated integrin activation (243).

1.3.5 Generation of microbicidal responses of macrophages

Triggering of respiratory burst in context of *Leishmania*-macrophage interaction

The characteristic feature of macrophages is the respiratory burst induced by phagocytosis, it reflects the activation of membrane-bound enzyme system NADPH-oxidase that transfers electrons from cytosolic NADPH to extracellular oxygen thereby producing superoxide ion (249). The oxidase is inactive in resting cells. In activated macrophages, *Leishmania* parasites are destroyed by synthesis of ROl (158). Perturbation of macrophages by the parasite may activate membrane-bound enzyme NADPH oxidase thereby catalysing the production of O_2^- from O_2. In orchestration and execution of the killing arms towards infection, macrophages initially encounter with the microorganisms, thereby triggering the generation of microbicidal metabolites through generation of O_2^-, oxygen-dependent killing mechanism. For the purpose of killing and immune response generation, ROl is involved (250); it is regarded as the first line of host defence during microbial invasion.

1.3.5.1 Production of reactive oxygen intermediates (ROI).

A drastic increase in oxygen consumption occurs following phagocytosis of microorganisms or any external stimuli by phagocytes (249, 251). As a result, superoxide (O_2^-) and hydrogen peroxide (H_2O_2), the oxygen metabolites were found to be introduced on greater amount (249). Microbial activity of phagocytes might be related to respiratory burst following phagocytosis (252). In the production of energy for the maintenance of host cell, products of the respiratory burst (O_2^- and H_2O_2) are probably not involved. Thus, they are involved in microbicidal activities of phagocytes. It is well known that there are three reactive forms of oxygen that may have microbicidal activity, formed during respiratory burst, viz, superoxide anion (O_2^-), Singlet ($^1O_2$) and hydroxyl radicals (OH) (253). The activated macrophages generate O_2^-, OH, H_2O_2 (140-144) which play key roles in killing of the *Leishmania* parasites.The series of biochemical events involved in the generation of reactive oxygen species are as follows:-

$$2O_2 + NADPH \xrightarrow{\text{Oxidase}} 2\,O_2^- + NADP^+ + H^+ \tag{1}$$

$$2O_2^- + 2H^+ \xrightarrow{\text{SOD}} O_2^- + H_2O_2 \tag{2}$$

$$2\,H_2O_2 \xrightarrow{\text{Catalase}} O_2 + H_2O \tag{3}$$

The first reaction occurs at the surface of the phagocytes or on the surface membrane invaginated into the phagosome (254). By an enzyme called NADPH oxidase, the oxygen is reduced to superoxide (255, 256). As a substrate, the NADPH is used which is produced in the Hexose monophosphate shunt. By the enzyme superoxide dismutase (SOD), superoxide is further reduced to H_2O_2, which is secreted inside the phagocyte vacuole. H_2O_2 is reduced by catalase to O_2 and to H_2O_2. Myeloperoxidase (MPO) is released into the vacuole, when the phagosomes containing the microorganisms fuse with lysosomes. H_2O_2 may react with O_2 forming Singlet oxygen ($^1O_2$), hydroxyl ion (OH) and hydroxyl radical (OH).

$$O_2^- + H_2O_2 \rightarrow OH^- + OH + {}^1O_2$$

These reactive forms of oxygen show microbicidal activity. The action of superoxide or Singlet oxygen could be that of lipid peroxidation that in turn inactivates enzymes or cross link proteins (257).

1.3.5.2 Production of reactive Nitrogen intermediates (RNI).

Nitric oxide (NO) acts as an important bioregulatory medium, performs many physiological functions. Nitric oxide and RNI are cytostatic and cytotoxic against tumor cells, generated by activated murine macrophages (258). These are also cytotoxic against intracellular and extracellular pathogens (259). NO is generated from the oxidation of the terminal guanido nitrogen atoms of L-arginine by NADPH dependent enzyme, NO synthases (NOS) (260), L-citruline is also generated from L-arginine. Important NOS activity inducers in murine macrophages are LPS, IFN-γ, TNF-α or migration inhibitory factor (260).

NO degrade as NO2- & NO3- :

$$H_2N\text{-}C\ (^+NH_2)NH - CH_2CH_2CH(^+NH_3) - COO^- + O_2 \rightarrow$$

$$NH_2CONH_2 - CH_2CH_2CH_2CH\ (^+NH_3) - COO^- + NO$$

$$2NO + O_2 \rightarrow 2NO_2$$

$$2NO_2 + H_2O \rightarrow NO_2^- + NO_3^- + 2H^+$$

Toxic effect of NO depends partly on cooperation with reactive O_2 intermediates. Interaction with nitric oxides causes nonheme iron associated with sulphur atoms to form nitrosyl-iron-sulphur complexes, resulting in iron loss from critical target enzymes and thereby causing metabolic failure of intracellular parasites. NO plays a key factor in killing *Leishmania* (229, 146, 148, 149, 153). NO derived from L-arginine by the catalytic action of NO synthase (NOS) plays an important role in killing parasites (261, 250). In plasma membrane, NO circulates as S-nitrosothiols (262). Above all, by the reaction of NO with O_2^-, peroxinitrite ($ONOO^-$) is produced, which is highly cytotoxic (263).

1.3.6 Evasion strategies of Leishmania parasites

For establishment of *Leishmania* infection, the prerequisite is the transformation of ingested promastigotes in macrophage into nonmotile amastigotes (264). The fate of the intracellular parasites is dependent on the parasite species and immune response of the host. Elaborate strategies are displayed by the parasite that enable evasion of the host's defence system. The basic evasion mechanisms are:

1.3.6.1 Evasion from cytotoxic serum

By binding of the receptor, which usually helps in the lysis of the parasites, is utilized by *Leishmania* to facilitate its entry into their host cells, thereby mediating their attachment to receptor.

1.3.6.2 Inhibition of oxidative burst

Intracellular *Leishmania* inhibits the generation of oxidative burst metabolites in macrophages (264, 265). Acid phosphatase activity (266) and two surface molecules of *Leishmania* viz. LPG (180-182, 268) and gp63 (183-185) are potent inhibitors of oxidative burst.

1.3.6.3 Scavenging of oxidative metabolites

LPG, gp63 are capable of protecting *Leishmania* from intralysosomal microbicidal factors (266, 267). Also, parasite shows high activity of enzymes, glutathione peroxidase, SOD, catalase, etc. which can degrade toxic macrophage products (158).

1.3.6.4 Inactivation of lysosomal enzymes within phagolysosome

LPG is capable of inhibiting lysosomal β-galactosidase (186, 188) and transmission of virulence to mammals (268). gp63 inactivates proteolytic host enzymes and protects parasite proteins from phagolysosomal degradation (266).

1.3.6.5 Inhibition of NO and cytokine production

Cytokines IFN-γ and TNF-α are secreted by activated macrophages to generate ROl and RNI for antiparasitic activity (144-149, 151, 152, 154- 159). *Leishmania* manipulates the host immune responses in order to protect itself and to gain entry into the cell. The unique adaptive mechanisms help promote Leishmanial survival inside the macrophage. This includes inhibition of NO and cytokine production (267, 229).

1.3.6.6 Macrophage cell signalling during interaction with *L.donovani* parasites

It is now known that during *Leishmania*-macrophage interaction, some definite sequential events occur as such attachment of the parasite to host cell leads to entry and uptake followed by multiplication. During attachment of various microorganisms with macrophages or other host cells following interaction activates PTK or PKC-mediated cell signalling molecules, as in *Salmonella typhimurium* (293), *Yersinia* sp. (119, 294), *E.coli* (295) and in *Streptococcus pyrogens* (385). These cells signalling molecules finally help in the internalisation of the pathogen. However during *Leishmania* attachment, these type of cell signalling (PTK and PKC) and resulting phosphorylating molecules are not studied. Although, after internalisation and during multiplication *Leishmania* survives long time within the macrophage by avoiding triggering of oxidative burst by impairing the oxidative responses of cells (272) and inhibits NO release (267, 271). The unique adaptive mechanisms help promote *Leishmania* survival by inhibiting macrophage cell signalling pathways (267, 237-239, 228, 229).

1.4 Therapeutic advances: problems and progress

1.4.1 Key factors hindering the search of antileishmanial agents.

Strains: There are about 20 different *Leishmania* species phenetic complex (Table 1A). Of these, *L. donovani* phenetic complex is found in more than one country. All *Leishmania* species exhibit similar morphology. Clinical, biological and serological tests often overlap and thus distinction between species is still not clear (10).

Look alike-amastigote: All amastigotes in vertebrate tissues look similar. They are spheroid to ovoid, usually 2-5μm to 5.0μm wide, some are though smaller. Insufficient information regarding the metabolism of the amastigotes is available.

Life cycle of the parasite: The most baffling problems in immunology presented by the life cycle of *Leishmania* species are:

The parasites in the vertebrate body live inside the macrophage (the unique cell, functions to kill invading organism). Within macrophage, the parasite resides and proliferates inside the phagolysosomes (the compartment meant for digesting foreign particles).

Clinical manifestations: In clinical manifestation, *Leishmania* species markedly differ with respect to infections ranging from self healing cutaneous one to fatal visceral one with extremely disfiguring afflictions which may disrupt regular facial features.

Human Genetic make-up and Nutritional State: The contributions of human host genetic make up and nutritional state to the course of infection have yet to be completely described in terms of handling Leishmaniasis immunology. Their complex and diverse host-parasitic interaction kept occupied the Leishmaniacs (Scientists involved in *Leishmania* research) for a long time.

Drug treatment precipitation: As in the case of PKDL (Post kala-azar dermal leishmanoid), in a subsequent clinical manifestation, the drug treatment may precipitate where original infection is quite different from the subsequent infection.

Serodiagnostic problem: These problems are based on:

a)   Problems which are asymmetric,

b)   Problem of detection that shows positive with previous infections,

c)   Problem that shows positive after treatment

Serodiagnostic methods based on RIA or ELISA which are followed in India for visceral Leishmaniasis often show cross-reactivity with other protozoal and bacterial diseases and are not very specific due to complex mixture of antigens. Though these problems are now quite checked by improved techniques of antigen purification, antigen polymerisation and antigen selection by monoclonal antibodies (36).

Drug limitations: All presently used drugs have limitations. Visceral Leishmaniasis is often resistant to pentamidine. Antimonials are too toxic on long time treatment and report of being resistant towards visceral form (37). After exposure to these drugs the disease relapses and PKDL may follow insufficient treatment. The second line of drug Amphotericin B (273) is too toxic to be used as first line of drug.

1.4.2 Therapeutics against *Leishmania*

1.4.2.1 Conventional therapeutic advances

The modern development of antimony therapy began from 1907 following experimental work of Plimmers and Thomson (274). The most effective antileishmanial agents (Table lF) are on clinical trials. The first and second line drugs used are all toxic and methods are now being developed to deliver drugs *in situ* so as to reduce their toxicity. According to the report of TDR (37), the cases resistant to most frequent used drugs (antimonials), are reaching alarming levels, produce side effects and refractory cases.

The second line of drugs as Amphotericin B and pentamidines are too toxic (273). Thus, in addition to use these conventional drugs, development of new therapeutics based on modulation of receptor and signalling events is necessary to control the disease. Table 1C shows the conventional drugs.

TABLE 1F: Examples of Compounds in Clinical Trials or under experimental investigation

Compound	Origin	Status	Disease
Imofosine	Boehringer Mannheim	In clinical trials for cancer. Trials for visceral Leishmaniasis in planning stage	Visceral Leishmaniasis Possibly cutaneous Leishmaniasis and Chagas disease
Lipid associated amphotericin B (LAAMB)	Vestar Inc.	In clinical trials	Visceral and mucosal Leishmaniasis
Allopurinol	Welcome	In clinical trials. Alone for Chagas disease and +/- antimony for Leishmaniasis	Leishmaniasis and Chagas disease
Paramomycin / Aminosidine	Farmitalia	Topical formulation (paramomycin) in clinical trial. Trials for systemic administration (aminosidine) in planning stage	Leishmaniasis
Sterol biosynthesis Inhibitors	Janssen, Sandoz, Merck and Bristol-Meyers-Squibb	Anti-fungal azoles in clinical trial. Other inhibitors under experimental investigation	Leishmaniasis and Chagas disease
SAM decarboxylase inhibitors; HETA types	Marion MerrellDow, Ciba-Geigy Roswell Park and academic Institutions	Experimental work encouraging May require admixture with DEMO	African trypanosomiasis including arsenic resistant T.b. rhodesiense

1.4.2.2 Immunotherapeutic advancement

In both innate and adaptive immune responses of different cell types, cytokines play an important role in immunoregulation. One of the principal cytokines that activate macrophages for enhanced killing of a variety of intracellular pathogens including *Leishmania*, interferon gamma (IFN-γ) play a great role (275). To study the growth of intracellular parasites, cytokines are used. Macrophage derived reactive nitrogen intermediates (RNI) or reactive oxygen intermediates (ROl) are the effector molecules associated with the killing of parasites. It has been also noted that cytokine-activated macrophages produce tumor necrosis factor (TNF-α) that eliminate *L.donovani* in humans (153). By using IFN-γ and TNF-α, a synergistic effect occurs that is associated with eradication of the parasite. The effector molecules associated with the killing of the parasites are macrophage-derived RNI and ROl.

1.4.2.3 Signal transduction based therapeutic advances

We know Protein kinases and phosphatases mediated phosphorylation and dephosphorylation regulate various functions of cell. Abnormal phosphorylation in the cells may cause various kinds of diseases including cancer, sepsis, multiple sclerosis (386, 387). Therefore, approaches are now being taken to design and synthesize various kinds of inhibitors to control the abnormal growth and cure. Inhibitors of PTK, Tyrphostin (303), genistein (302) are now in market. In case of *Leishmania*, different receptors are exploited for cell signalling-mediated therapeutic approaches (276, 331). Efforts are now being made to manipulate the signalling cascade in such a way so as to inhibit disease progression. As a new therapeutic approach, the inhibitors of different important enzymes in signalling cascades for the production of ROI and RNI are now being stressed (230, 277-279) for many important diseases. Work on this signalling-based therapeutic approach can open new avenues in combating this deadly disease.

Scope of the present study

Despite all efforts on chemotherapy, till date visceral Leishmaniasis caused by *Leishmania donovani* still remains fatal and widespread. As an intramacrophage pathogen, the parasite is most successful in exploiting the host cell metabolism, targeting the host protein into phagolysosomal compartment and modulating its phagosome. Even today, because of the complexity of the disease antileishmanial therapy is an incomprehensible subject. The ground reality is that very few agents have adequately been assessed in clinical trials and the most effective agents have the most potential toxic effects and are difficult to administer. As alternative approach, people are now trying to exploit several surface receptors of host cells, e.g., macrophages for activation purposes to fight against this deadly pathogen, *L.donovani*. We therefore, thought that attempt could be made to control leishmanial infection either by modulating the surface receptor of macrophage or by identifying the signalling molecules generated say, kinases during early phases of *L.donovani*-macrophage i.e., ligand-receptor interaction. Identifying these types of molecules would help one to design suitable inhibitors for blocking the infections.

Although interaction of *L. donovani* with macrophages is known to be a ligand-receptor interaction, various aspects of macrophage surface receptor biology including:

i] modulation of receptors and its effect on the interaction process and ii] receptor signalling involving cell-cell interaction at the surface remains totally untouched. Work on this area will help us to understand the mechanism of controlling the infections and of intracellular survival of this pathogen.

INTERACTION OF *LEISHMANIA DONOVANI* WITH MODULATED MANNOSE RECEPTOR OF MACROPHAGE AND CONTROL OF LEISHMANIAL INFECTION

2

2.1 Introduction

The mannose receptor is well characterised on the surface of mature macrophages and is thought to play an important role in the recognition of mannose-containing glycoconjugates and in clearing lysosomal enzymes from the extracellular space (209). Expression of this receptor on the cell surface can be modulated by a variety of agents. Receptor expression is increased by treatment with dexamethasone (209) and vitamin D (210), whereas treatment with swainsonine (211), interferon (IFN-γ) (108), and H_2O_2 (212) decreases expression. Physiological studies indicate that this receptor may partcipate in a variety of functions involving both up- and down-regulation of expression.

Leishmania donovani, the causative agent of visceral Leishmaniasis, or kala-azar, is an obligate intracellular parasite that survives within the phagolysosomes of its hosts' macrophages. Several studies conducted on intact parasites have implicated a variety of receptors that may function in the binding of the promastigote form of the parasites to macrophages. These include the mannose receptor (177), a receptor of advanced glycosylation end products (AGE) (280), and the types 1 and 3 complement receptors (CR1, CR3) (121, 124, 126).

Macrophages are known to play a major role in host responses at sites of inflammation. Oxidants are a prominent constituent of the inflammatory milieu, and glucocorticoids are used extensively as anti-inflammatory agents; these agents are important modulators of mannose receptor activity. The present study was undertaken to investigate whether *in vitro* modulation of the macrophage mannose receptor by these agents affects the attachment and internalisation of virulent and avirulent *L. donovani* promastigotes.

2.2 Materials and Methods

2.2.1 Media and chemicals

RPMI 1640, bovine serum (FBS, heat inactivated) were from Difco (Detroit, Michigan); M199, penicillin, streptomycin, and gentamycin were from Gibco Laboratories (Grand Island, New York), Dexamethasone, p-NH$_2$-phenyl-α-D-mannopyranoside, bovine serum albumin (BSA), catalase, and glucose oxidase were from Sigma Chemical Co. (St. Louis, Missouri). All other reagents used were of analytical grade.

2.2.2 Parasites

Leishmania donovani strain UR6 (MHOM/lN/1978/UR6) (281) was isolated from an Indian patient with kala-azar. The organisms were maintained and grown in modified Ray's medium (282) and subcultures were made at 72-hr intervals, *L.donovani* AG83 (MHOM/IN/1983/AG83) and GE-I (MHOM/IN/89/GE-l) strains were maintained in female BALB/c mice. Parasites were recovered from the spleen of infected mice by adding spleens to culture medium (M199 supplemented with 20% FBS, 100U/mI penicillin, and 100µg/ml streptomycin). The cultures were kept for 5 days at 22°C to obtain the promastigotes, which were then washed and used for infection of macrophages.

2.2.3 Preparation of macrophages

Macrophages were prepared as previously described (283). Briefly, thioglycollate-elicited macrophages were isolated by peritoneal lavage from female Swiss albino mice. Cells were plated in 35-mm tissue culture plates for 2 hr at 37°C. The cells were washed extensively with phosphate-buffered saline (PBS) (20 mM sodium phosphate buffer containing 0.15 M NaCI, pH7.4) to remove any nonadherent cells. Cells obtained this way were ~85% viable, as judged by trypan blue exclusion test.

2.2.4 Treatment of macrophages with oxidants or dexamethasone

Medium was removed from the cells on cover slips and replaced with fresh medium containing oxidant or oxidant-generating system with or without catalase (100µg/ml) or dexamethasone, and incubated at 37°C with H$_2$O$_2$ (0.25 – 1.0 min) for 30 min, glucose (10 mM) plus glucose oxidase (500 µg /mI) for 30 min, and dexamethasone; a stock solution of dexamethasone was made in absolute ethanol as described elsewhere (209). Dilutions were made before use in PBS and added to cultures as 0.1 – 0.2 µg/ml for 20 hr.

2.2.5 Infection of macrophages

Promastigote forms of the parasites were used to infect cultures of adherent macrophages at a ratio of 10 parasites per macrophage. Infection was allowed to proceed for 2 hr at 37°C; then all extracellular parasites were washed out. In most instances, 80% of the macrophages were infected. Infection levels were determined by microscopic examination of Giemsa stained cells.

2.2.6 Preparation of mannose-BSA and AGE-BSA

Mannose-BSA (Man-BSA) was prepared according to the method previously described (284). Briefly, p-aminophenyl-α-D-mannopyranoside was coupled to BSA through water-soluble 1-ethyl-3-(3-dimethyl aminopropyl)-carbodiimide hydrochloride at pH 4.75. After coupling, sugar and protein were estimated by phenol-sulphuric acid (285) and Lowry methods (286), respectively.

For the mannose receptor blocking experiment with Man-BSA, macrophages were incubated in the absence or presence of H_2O_2 (500 μM) or dexamethasone (0.1 μgm/ml) at 37°C, washed, and Man-BSA was added to both treated and untreated macrophages. Both virulent and avirulent parasites were then added and incubated at 37°C for 2 hr.

AGE-BSA was prepared by incubating protein solution (BSA, 25 mg/ml) with 0.5 mM glucose in 0.15 M phophate buffer, pH 7.3, at 37°C for 4 weeks in the presence of 1.5 mM phenylmethylsulfonyl fluoride (PMSF), 0.5mM EDTA, penicillin (100 μg/ml), and gentamycin (40 μg/ml) under sterile conditions according to the method of Vlassara et al (287). After incubation, low molecular-weight reactants were removed by dialysis against PBS. Sugar and protein were then analysed again as described above. Both ligands were iodinated using a chloramine-T procedure (288).

2.2.7 Binding of ^{125}I-Man-BSA, ^{125}I-AGE-BSA by mouse peritoneal macrophages

Binding studies were performed with peritoneal macrophages in α-MEM plus 10% FBS buffered with 20 mM 3-(Nmorpholino) propanesulfonic acid (MOPS), adjusted to pH 7.0. Adherent macrophage cells were first scraped with a disposable cell scraper and were suspended in the binding medium, washed twice with the medium cooled to 4°C, and incubated for 2 hr with radioiodinated ligands (5×10^5 counts per minute) in the presence or absence of 100-fold excess of unlabeled cold ligands or mannan (2 mg/ml). After incubation, the cells were washed extensively, solubilized, and assayed for radioactivity in a γ-radiation counter. The protein was estimated by the Lowry procedure (286).

2.2.8 Effect of H_2O_2 or dexamethasone treatment on attachment and uptake of parasites

Macrophages were incubated with H_2O_2 or dexamethasone for 30 min or 20 hr. The cells were washed extensively with PBS and then incubated with virulent or avirulent *L. donovani* promastigotes. After incubation, the excess promastigotes were removed and the cells were washed with PBS. Cells were then air-dried, fixed, stained with Giemsa, and the number of attachment and internalised parasites counted using light microscopy.

2.3 Results

2.3.1 Effects of H_2O_2 or dexamethasone on mannose receptor activity of peritoneal macrophage cells

Binding of ^{125}I-Man-BSA (ligand) to mannose receptor of macrophages is shown in Figure 2.1. Macrophages were pre-treated with increasing concentrations of H_2O_2 for 30 min at 37°C or with dexamethasone for 20 hr. More than half-maximal inhibition in binding was achieved with 500 μM H_2O_2 with maximal effects at 1 mM H_2O_2 (Fig.2.1A). In contrast, treatment with dexamethasone shows a near 2-fold increase in cell surface binding at 0.1μg/ml (Fig.2.1B). Although it was reported that 1 mM H_2O_2 had no effect on macrophage viability (212), little toxicity was observed at this concentration in which 80-85% of cells excluded trypan blue.

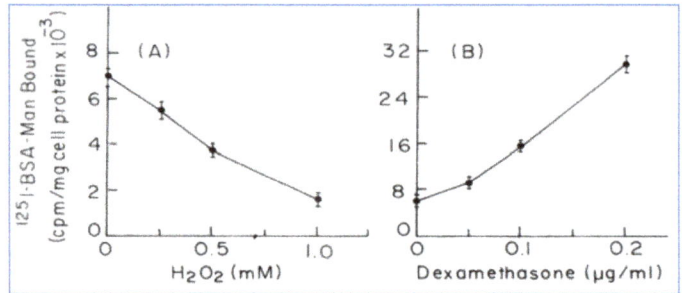

FIG. 2.1:   Effects of H_2O_2 or dexamethasone on binding of ^{125}I-mannose-bovine serum albumin (^{125}I-MAN-BSA).

A. Effects of H_2O_2 treatment at 37°C on binding of ^{125}I-MAN-BSA. Mouse peritoneal macrophages were incubated in the presence or absence of H_2O_2 at 37°C for 30 min, cooled, washed and resuspended in assay medium at 10^7 cells/ml. Control and H_2O_2- treated cells were incubated at 4°C with 5 x 10^5 counts/min. of ^{125}I-MAN-BSA for 2 hr. Cells were collected and radioactivity quantified.

B. Effect of dexamethasone on binding of ^{125}I-MAN-BSA. Macrophages were cultured and dexamethsone was added at the concentration indicated. At the end of incubation, the cells were washed and ^{125}I-MAN-BSA was added. Cells were collected and radioactivity quantified as in A.

2.3.2 Effect of H_2O_2 or dexamethasone on phagocytic activities of peritoneal macrophages for *L. donovani* strains

As a mannose receptor of macrophages is involved in the recognition of *L.donovani* promastigotes, an attempt was made to evaluate the contribution of this receptor after treatment with H_2O_2 or dexamethasone toward the uptake of virulent and avirulent strains of *L. donovani* promastigotes. In general, H_2O_2 exerted an inhibitory effect on the uptake of parasites (Fig.2.2) the inhibition was maximum for the avirulent strain (UR6), i.e. about 45%, whereas for virulent strains (AG-83) and (GE-I), inhibition was roughly 30 and 25%, respectively. However, dexamethasone stimulated macrophages to take up the parasites. Again, for the avirulent strain, maximum stimulation in uptake was at least 3 times greater compared with the untreated control.

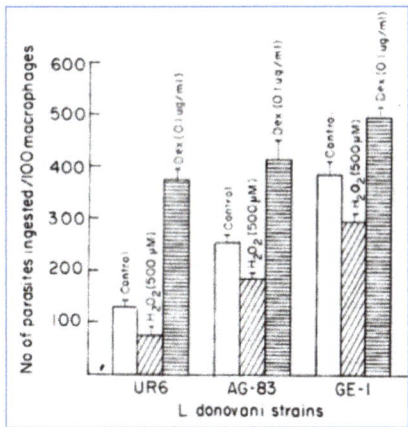

FIG. 2.2: Effect of H_2O_2 or dexamethasone on mannose receptor mediated uptake of *Leishmania donovani* strains by mouse peritoneal macrophages. Cells were incubated in absence or presence of H_2O_2 or dexamethasone and washed and promastigotes were added, washed and counted for uptake by light microscopy.

2.3.3 H_2O_2 mediated *L.donovani* promastigote uptake by mannose receptor: block by catalase

Since maximal inhibition in uptake of avirulent parasites (UR6) was observed by H_2O_2-treated macrophages, an effort was made to examine whether the actual decrease in mannose receptor, or indirectly the inhibition in uptake of UR6, was due to the effect of H_2O_2. For this, macrophages were coincubated with H_2O_2 and catalase (100 µg/ml) for 30 min at 37°C, washed, and then charged with UR6. Coincubation of H_2O_2 and catalase blocked the inhibition of uptake.

2.3.4 Effect of artificially generated oxidant system on attachment and uptake of *L. donovani* promastigotes

Glucose-plus glucose oxidase, capable of artificially generating reactive oxygen species, was examined to study their effects on the uptake of UR6 and AG83 promastigotes. It is known that 500mU of glucose oxidase produces 100 nmol/ml of H_2O_2 per minute (212). When macrophages were pretreated with 500 µg/ml of glucose oxidase, there was 40% inhibition in attachment and 42% in internalisation for UR6, and 24% inhibition in attachment and 30% in internalisation for AG83 (Table 2A).

TABLE 2A: Effect of artificial H_2O_2 generating system (glucose+glucose oxidase) on the attachment and uptake of *Leishmania donovani* promastigotes1

	Control		H_2O_2		Glucose+glucose oxidase	
L.donovani						
Stains[2]	**Attachment**	**Internalisation**	**Attachment**	**Internalisation**	**Attachment**	**Internalisation**
UR6	202 ± 7.0	143 ± 6.0	130 ± 6.0	90 ± 3.0	122 ± 4.0	85 ± 7.0
AG83	78 ± 6.0	264 ± 9.0	50 ± 9.0	175 ± 5.0	59 ± 8.0	187 ± 10.0

[1]Data shown are the mean ±S.D (n=3)
[2]Macrophages were treated for 30 min with 10 mM glucose plus 30µg/ml of glucose oxidase.

TABLE 2B: Effect of H_2O_2 or dexamethasone on advanced glycosylation end product (AGE) receptor of macrophages[1]

Treatment	^{125}I-Bovine serum albumin (BSA)-AGE bound to macrophages (cpm)		
	(-) Cold AGE-BSA	(+) Cold AGE-BSA	Specific binding
None	8,395 ± 148.0	4,275 ± 106.0	4,120
H_2O_2 (500 µM)	8,262 ± 88.0	4,415 ± 49.0	3,847
Dexamethasone (0.1 µg/ml)	8,712 ± 123.0	4,482 ± 130.0	4,230

[1]These data are representative of 3 separate experiments. Results are expressed as the mean ± S.D.

2.3.5 Effect of H_2O_2 or dexamethasone on other macrophage receptors

To examine the effect of oxidant or dexamethasone treatment on other macrophage receptors, binding of another ligand by another macrophage receptor (AGE receptor) was measured. Incubation of macrophages with H_2O_2 or dexamethasone decreased or increased mannose receptor-mediated binding of ^{125}I-Man-BSA, whereas binding of ^{125}I-AGE-BSA on AGE receptor of macrophages was virtually unaffected (90% of control) (Table 2B). To determine indirectly that the expression of both CR1 and CR3 are not affected after the modification of macrophage surface by H_2O_2 or dexamethasone, mannose receptors of macrophage were blocked with freshly prepared Man-BSA. Macrophages were then challenged with both virulent and avirulent strains of *L.donovani* promastigotes and their uptake was studied (Table 2C). It is obvious that the uptake did not change before and after the treatment with H_2O_2 or dexamethasone, showing indirectly that the macrophage surface modification does not involve all the receptors.

TABLE-2C: Effect of H2O2 or dexamethasone on macrophage noncarbohydrate receptor-mediated uptake of virulent or avirulent *Leishmania donovani* promastigote1

Cells + treatment	No. of parasites/ 100 macrophages
Macrophage + UR6	144 ± 5.0
Macrophage + Man-BSA + UR6	63 ± 3.0
Macrophage + H_2O_2 + UR6	94 ± 3.0
Macrophage + H_2O_2 + Man-BSA + UR6	68 ± 6.0
Macrophage + dex. + UR6	361 ± 9.0
Macrophage + dex. + Man-BSA + UR6	73 ± 5.0
Macrophage + AG-83	252 ± 11.0
Macrophage + Man-BSA + AG-83	149 ± 6.0
Macrophage + H_2O_2 + AG-83	168 ± 7.0
Macrophage + H_2O_2 + Man-BSA + AG-83	138 ± 4.0
Macrophage + dex. + AG-83	411 ± 13.0
Macrophage + dex. + Man-BSA + AG-83	163 ± 5.0
Macrophage + GE-1	376 ± 8.0
Macrophage + Man-BSA + GE-1	244 ± 3.0
Macrophage + H_2O_2 + GE-1	213 ± 3.0
Macrophage + H_2O_2 + Man-BSA + GE-1	236 ± 3.0
Macrophage + dex. + GE-1	472 ± 7.0
Macrophage + dex. + Man-BSA + GE-1	241 ± 8.0

[1]These data are representative of 3 separate experiments. Results are expressed as mean ± S.D. Man-BSA, mannose-bovine serum albumin; dex., dexamethasone; UR6, avirulent strain; AG-83 and GE-I, virulent strains.

2.4 Discussion

Macrophages have been shown to play a major role in host responses at sites of inflammation. Oxidants generated at the inflammatory sites and the anti-inflammatory agent used *in vivo* are known to regulate mannose receptor activity of macrophages *in vitro*. Mannose receptors may participate in a variety of physiologic functions involving both up and down regulation of receptor expression, as, for example, expression of this receptor is low in macrophages that have been activated to a tumoricidal state (51, 57). In the present study, an effort was made to determine whether and to what extent specific inhibition of mannose receptor activity by oxidants or up regulation of the same receptor by anti-inflammatory steroid, dexamethasone, affect the attachment and internalisation of virulent and avirulent *L.donovani* promastigotes. Macrophages have a variety of receptors on their cell surface, including the mannose receptor, which mediates the uptake of *L. donovani* promastigotes. In the present study, H_2O_2 and dexamethasone were shown to differentially affect mannose receptor-mediated attachment and internalisation of virulent and avirulent strains by peritoneal macrophages. It is known that H_2O_2 down regulates and dexamethasone up regulates the expression of the mannose receptor (209, 212). A similar result was seen in the binding experiment of ^{125}I-Man-BSA with H_2O_2 or dexamethasone-treated cells (Fig.2.1A, 2.1B). In H_2O_2 treated cells, inhibition in uptake was greater for avirulent strains compared with the virulent ones (Fig. 2.2). In contrast, in dexamethasone treated macrophages, uptake was enhanced for avirulent strains in comparison with virulent strains. These results clearly indicate that H_2O_2 and dexamethasone have opposite effects on the uptake of parasites via the mannose receptor of macrophages and that the avirulent strain used this receptor more efficiently. This decrease or increase in uptake was probably due to a decrease or increase in the binding of promastigotes, which is in close agreement with previous results (95, 289), where it was shown that virulent strains use CR3 and avirulent strains use the mannosyl fucosyl receptor for their maximum uptake. In a similar approach, Mosser and Handman (290) reported that IFN-γ treated macrophages bind fewer *L. major* and *L. donovani* promastigotes than untreated cells because of down regulation of a lectin-like receptor. In addition to H_2O_2, glucose/glucose oxidase which enzymatically generates H_2O_2, decreased the uptake of the parasites and the decrease was blocked by catalase (Table 2A). The above result suggests that the artificially generating oxidant system behaved similarly to H_2O_2. There was no cell death after treatment with 500 μM of H_2O_2 for 30 min or with dexamethasone (0.1μg/ml) for 20 hr as assessed by trypan blue exclusion and the protein content of adherent macrophages.

It might be possible that treatment of macrophages with H_2O_2 or dexamethasone would affect other macrophage receptors. Binding of ligands by the AGE receptor (287) was not affected by treatment with H_2O_2 or dexamethasone. The results also showed, though indirectly, that both CR1 and CR3 are not affected by these treatments. Thus, the modulation by H_2O_2 or dexamethasone at these levels appears to be selective for the mannose receptor.

INTERACTION OF *LEISHMANIA DONOVANI* WITH MACROPHAGE AND ACTIVATION OF PROTEIN TYROSINE KINASE

3

3.1 Introduction

Leishmania donovani, the intracellular protozoan which causes visceral Leishmaniasis or kala-azar in humans, selectively parasitizes resident macrophages within the liver, the spleen, and the bone marrow. The *Leishmania*-macrophage interaction is known to be receptor-mediated and several studies indicated that a variety of receptors on the surface of the host cell may function in the binding of the promastigote form of the parasites to macrophages. These receptors include the integrin receptors CR1 and CR3, mannose receptor and a receptor for advanced glycosylation end products (124, 121, 280).

Receptor ligation is accompanied by a localized rise in tyrosine phosphorylation, which can be mediated by different family of protein tyrosine kinases (226, 227). During ingestion of a particle or pathogen, under the influence of PTKs, different cytoskeleton proteins are recruited to the cytoplasmic face of membranes adjacent to particles and this alongwith the polymerisation of host cell actin, provide the necessary force to extend the pseudopodia around the particle and ingest it (291, 292). Although general understanding of the participation of PTKs in infectious diseases is incipient, considerable progress has been made in bacterial models. Tyrosine phosphorylation was observed during *Salmonella typhimurium* invasion into epithelial cells (293) and also, *Yersinia* sp (119, 294) and *Escherichia coli* (295) entry induces tyrosine phosphorylation of specificproteins involved in cytoskeletal rearrangement. To activate the cytoskeletal rearrangement necessary for the uptake of pathogens, the receptor-ligand interaction between host and pathogen must induce signal to target the actin. Ligand binding to integrin, FyR1 and CR3 receptors of host cells have recently been demonstrated to send signals to the cytoskeleton (296-298).

Protein tyrosine phosphorylation and dephosphorylation controls various functions of host-pathogen interaction and are controlled by the concerted action of PTKs and phosphatases. Although, antigens isolated from various parasitic protozoa were shown to induce PTK activity on mammalian cells (299-301), little is known about the PTK signaling events associated with invasion by living protozoa. In this study, we investigated the involvement of PTKs and phosphatases in the uptake and intracellular replication of virulent and avirulent *Leishmania donovani* promastigotes in macrophages. Furthermore, we examined whether the PTK activation signals are necessary to induce the cytoskeletal rearrangement required for the entry of parasites and the possibility that these signals differ between avirulent and virulent parasites during intracellular replication of this pathogen.

3.2 Materials and Methods

3.2.1 Media and Chemicals

Medium 199, RPMI 1640, Fetal bovine serum, penicillin, streptomycin and gentamycin were from GIBCO Laboratories, Grand Island, NY, USA. Chemicals, tyrphostin 25, genistein, cytochalasin B, N-1-napthylethylenediamine dihydrochloride and sodium orthovanadate were from Sigma Chemical Co., St. Louis, MO. All other reagents used were of analytical grade.

3.2.2 Parasites

Pathogenic strains of *Leishmania donovani*, GE-1 (MHOM/IN/89/GE-1) and AG-83 (MHOM/IN/1983/AG 83) were used in this study. Amastigote form of the parasites were isolated from the spleen of the infected BALB/c mice which had been infected 6-8 weeks earlier. Freshly transformed virulent promastigote form of the parasites were obtained from amastigotes by culturing them into M199 supplemented with 20% heat-inactivated fetal bovine serum (FBS), 0.15M Hepes, 100 µg penicillin and 100 µg streptomycin/ml. Promastigotes population were maintained at 22°C and harvested during the stationary growth phase. Non-pathogenic strain UR6 (MHOM/lN/1978/UR6) was maintained in solid blood agar medium at 22°C and subcultures were made after 72 hrs (281).

3.2.3 Macrophages

Mouse peritoneal macrophages were isolated from the peritoneal cavity of BALB/c mice after 4 days of the intraperitoneal injection of 1 ml of sodium thioglycollate (4%) as described previously (239). Briefly, the cells were plated on glass coverslips and allowed to adhere for 2 hr at 37°C at 5% CO_2 atmosphere, after which the non-adhering cells were removed by extensive washing with PBS and fresh culture medium (RPMI 1640 plus 10% FBS) added.

3.2.4 Infection of macrophage cells

For infection, washed promastigotes, virulent or avirulent and macrophages were left in contact for 1 hr at 35°C in a parasite: macrophage ratio of 20:1 in medium RPMI

1640. After the incubation, the cells were washed at least three times with PBS to remove unbound parasites from the monolayer. Infection levels were determined by microscopic examination of at least 200 to 300 Giemsa-stained cells on each coverslip and the experiments were repeated at least three times.

3.2.5 Inhibition or augmentation assays with PTK and PTPase antagonists

Macrophage monolayers were incubated with tyrosine kinase inhibitors genistein for 30 min or with tyrphostin-25, 45 min prior to parasite infection. Genistein (302) restricts ATP binding, while tyrphostin (303) inhibits substrate binding to the catalytic domain of the PTKs. Number of parasites/100 macrophages was determined by counting 500 to 1000 inhibitor-treated or non-treated cells.

To determine the effects of drugs on intracellular parasite replication, cells were infected for 2 hr, and then treated with inhibitors. The cells were then washed and incubated again with the inhibitors for 2 hr, and fixed and stained at 12, 24 and 48 hrs to check the intracellular replication.

To test the effect of protein tyrosine phosphatase inhibitor, macrophages were infected with promastigotes for 60 min. in the presence or absence of different vanadate concentrations, or using both genistein and vanadate prior to 60 min infection with promastigotes.

3.2.6 Macrophages actin polymerization and Parasite phagocytosis assay

Inhibitor of actin polymerization, cytochalasin B, was used to study the role of f-actin in parasite phagocytosis. Cytochalasin B was diluted from a stock solution (1 mg/ml in DMSO) to 10 µg/mI into each coverslip. The cells were pretreated for 30-40 min, and the cytochalasin B was left in throughout the assay. As a control, equivalent amounts of vehicle (DMSO) were added to parallel monolayers. Macrophage monolayers were then incubated with virulent or avirulent promastigotes for approximately 1 hr, washed and then the number of organisms associated with the monolayer was determined by the microscopic examination of Giemsa-stained cells.

3.2.7 Nitrite determination during parasite replication

Nitrite accumulation in the culture supernatants of infected macrophages treated or non-treated with PTK inhibitors was determined as described previously (304). Briefly, 400 µl samples from 48 hr infected macrophages treated with IFN-γ/LPS were harvested and mixed with an equal volume of Griess reagent (0.5% sulfanilamide and 0.05%-N-1-napthylethylene diamine dihydrochloride in 50% phosphoric acid) at room temperature for 10 min. The absorbance was monitored spectrophotometrically at 550 nm against standards (sodium nitrite) in the same medium.

3.3 Results

3.3.1 Effect of PTK and PTPase antagonists on entry of virulent and avirulent *Leishmania donovani* promastigotes into macrophages

To study the contribution of PTKs in *Leishmania donovani* entry into macrophages, monolayers were pretreated with PTK inhibitors, genistein or tyrphostin prior to infection. Both the inhibitors decreased parasite entry in a dose-dependent manner. However, tyrphostin 25 was a more effective inhibitor of *Leishmania donovani* entry than was genistein (Fig.3A$_1$, 3A$_2$). A 45 min treatment of macrophages with 8 µM tyrphostin 25 prior to infection decreased invasion of two virulent strains GE-1 and AG-83 by 88% and 85% respectively, whereas for the avirulent strain UR6, the decrease in invasion was approximately 86%. Treatment with genistein at 400 µM for 30 min led to a decrease in invasion by 76% and 73% for GE-1 and AG-83 and 75% for the avirulent strain UR6. The concentrations of genistein and tyrphostin used in the experiment had no effect on host cell viability as measured by trypan blue dye exclusion. Thus PTK antagonists restricted *Leishmania donovani* promastigote invasion in a dose-dependent manner and the decrease in invasion was almost to a similar extent for both virulent and avirulent promastigotes.

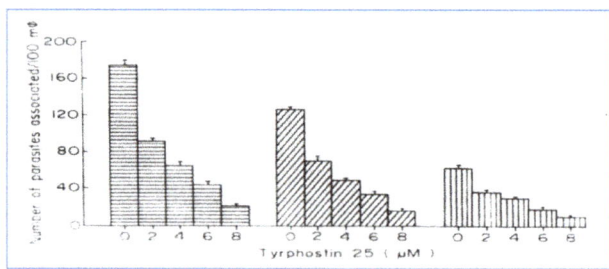

Fig.3A$_1$

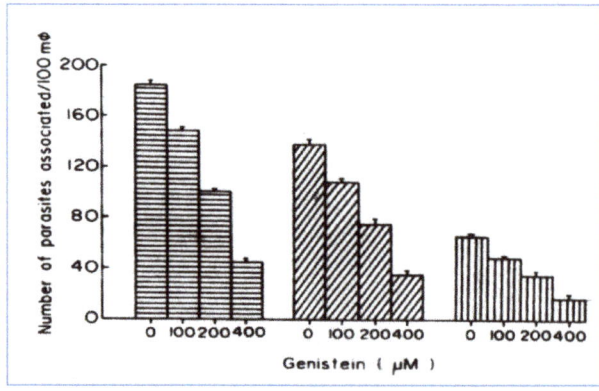

Fig.3A$_2$

FIG. 3A: Uptake inhibition studies with various strains of *L. donovani* infected macrophage (MØ) pretreated with PTK inhibitors, Tyrphostin 25 (3A1) and Genistein (3A2). MØ monolayers were prepared, preincubated with different kinase inhibitors at different concentrations and at different time points as described and then allowed to infect with either GE-1 ▦ strain or AG-83 ▨ or UR-6 ▥ for 1 hr. Results are mean of three different experiments performed with duplicate samples.

To determine the role of protein tyrosine phosphatase in the entry of parasites into macrophages, cells were pretreated with sodium orthovanadate, an inhibitor (305, 306) of tyrosine phosphatase. Addition of vanadate, prior to 60 min infection with promastigotes, increased the uptake in a dose dependent manner. At 250 μM of drug, there was almost 2-3 fold increase in uptake for the virulent strains GE-1 and AG-83 and slightly more than two folds for the avirulent strain UR6 (Fig.3C$_1$). However, when macrophages were coincubated with vanadate and PTK inhibitor genistein, the drug was able to partially revert genistein inhibition of *Leishmania* invasion (Fig 3C$_2$) indicating that protein tyrosine phosphorylation and dephosphorylation might have a definite role in the uptake of *Leishmania donovani* promastigotes.

3.3.2 Effect of PTK antagonists on intracellular replication of parasites

To test whether the PTK inhibitors affect the intracellular replication of *Leishmania donovani*, macrophage cells infected with GE-1 or AG-83 strains for 2 hr were treated with genistein or tyrphostin and intracellular survival and replication of parasites were assayed. As shown in Fig.3B, at 12 hr and 48 hr, the number of GE-1 parasites/100 macrophages was 375±7.5 and 1194± 13.0 in untreated control, whereas with 8μM tyrpohostin-25 or with 400 μM genistein, the number of parasites/100 cells was 410±9.5 and 1146 ± 14.0 or 353±6.0 and 1218±10.9 respectively. Similarly, with AG-83 strain at 48 hr, the number of parasites in untreated control was 642±7.3 compared to 603±7.41 and 682± 4.40 with tyrphostin or genistein treated cells.

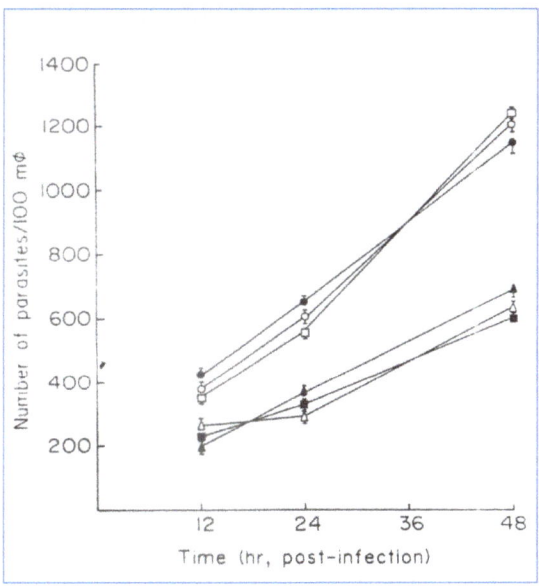

FIG. 3B: Effect of PTK inhibitors on intracellular replication of virulent strains of *L. donovani* promastigotes. MØ monolayers were infected with GE-1 or AG-83 strains for 2 hrs and then were treated with genistein (30min) and Tyrphostin 25 (1 hr) and then washed and kept for different times points (post-infected). Designated as untreated control GE-1 (o), GE-1 treated with Tyrphostin 25 (●) or Genistein (□) and untreated control AG-83 (■), AG-83 treated with Tyrphostin 25(Δ) or Genistein (▲). Results are mean ± S.D. of three separate experiments.

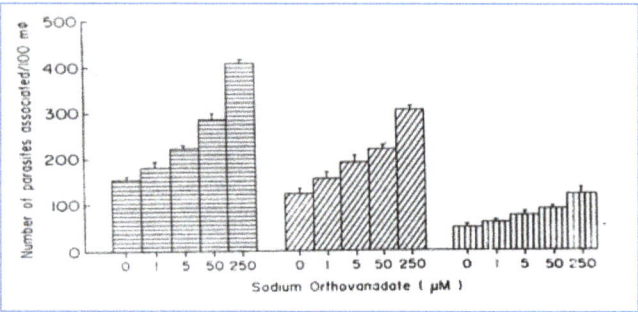

Fig.3C₁

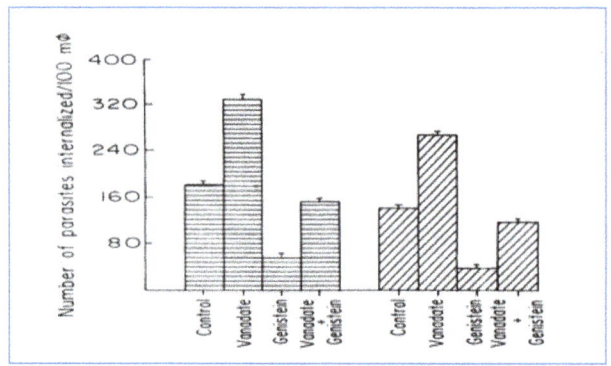

Fig.3C₂

FIG. 3C: Increased uptake of *Leishmania* promastigotes by macrophages induced by the protein tyrosine phosphatase inhibitor sodium orthovanadate (3C₁). Macrophages were infected with promastigotes, [GE-1 🔳 strain or AG-83 🔲 or UR-6🔲] for 1 hr in the presence or absence of different vanadate concentration (3C₂). Macrophages were incubated with 100 μM vanadate, 400 μM genistein or both drugs prior to 60 min infection with promastigotes. Data are mean ± S.D. of 3 independent experiments.

Collectively, these results indicated that neither genistein nor tyrphostin significantly reduced intracellular replication of *Leishmania donovani* in macrophages compared to untreated cells following 48 hrs of incubation. The inhibitors were also proved to be not lethal to intracellular pathogens if they were lethal, then the parasites should not replicate during the continued 48 hr of infection.

3.3.3 Macrophage actin polymerisation and phagocytosis of *Leishmania donovani* promastigotes

As PTK-mediated signal induces actin polymerization and actin polymerization affects in the phagocytosis of various bacterial models (307- 309), we next tried to examine whether cytochalasin B, an inhibitor of actin polymerization affects in the phagocytosis of *Leishmania donovani* promastigotes or not. Cytochalasin B treated or untreated macrophage cells were incubated with virulent or avirulent *Leishmania donovani* promastigotes for around 1 hr. The number of organisms associated with the monolayer and their cellular location was determined. Virulent promastigotes (GE-1 and AG- 83) bound avidly to both control and cytochalasin B-treated cells. In untreated macrophages, most of the cell-associated organisms were found inside however, virtually all of the parasites associated with parallel monolayers of cytochalasin-treated macrophages remained peripherally attached outside the cells (Table-3A). However, in case of avirulent strain UR6, all organisms were found attached on the macrophages in cytochalasin B-treated cells and as expected fewer organisms were found attached onto the surface of untreated cells, Thus, the inhibition in phagocytosis of *Leishmania donovani* promastigotes following treatment of macrophages with cytochalasin strongly suggested that actin signals and actin polymerization are necessary for the phagocytosis of promastigotes by macrophages.

TABLE - 3A: Effect of cytochalasin B on internalization of virulent or avirulent *L. donovani* promastigotes by mouse macrophages

Cell	Treatment[1]	*Leishmania* /100 macrophages Attached	Internalized
Macrophages + GE-1	Cytochalasin B	178 ± 2.13	15 ± 1.50
Macrophages + GE-1	---	---	182 ± 1.71
Macrophages + AG-83	Cytochalasin B	134 ± 2.91	17 ± 3.0
Macrophages + AG-83	--	---	148 ± 1.42
Macrophages + UR6	Cytochalasin B	70 ± 1.83	---
Macrophages + UR6	---	15 ± 2.50	65 ± 1.15

[1] Macrophages were pretreated with 10 μg/ml cytochalasin B and then parasites were added to be treated or untreated monolayers for 1 hr. Following 1-hr incubation, monolayers were washed, fixed, stained and examined under microscope. Results represent the mean of triplicate determinations ± S.D.

3.3.4 Correlation between nitric oxide production and *Leishmania* multiplication

Nitric oxide of macrophages is known to play a major role in both antibacterial and antiparasitic activity (310, 145). In order to understand the role and status of NO during intracellular replication of *Leishmania* parasites, NO was determined both in control infected and PTK inhibitors-treated infected macrophages. At 48 hr after infection with GE-1 parasites, the level of NO_2^- was 29.6±1.71 μ moles/10^6 cells, compared to 36.3±1.60 μ moles with tyrphostin and 34.6±1.71 μ moles with genistein (Table-3B). On the other hand, at the same time point with AG-83 parasites, NO_2^- levels were 40.33±2.20 μ moles in control infected macrophages compared to 43.66±1.11 μ moles and 49±1.0 μ moles for tryphostin and genistein treated cells respectively. This result is in agreement with previous report that NO plays an important role in regulation of leishmanial infection. Thus, in our replication study, PTK inhibitors could not inhibit the NO production significantly and hence the multiplication.

3.4 Discussion

Protein kinases and phosphatases are known to play important roles in various kinds of cell-cell interaction, e.g. cell adhesion, internalization and killing of pathogens

TABLE - 3B: Effect of PTK inhibitors on nitric oxide production during parasite multiplication

Cells	Treatment[1]	Nitrite[2] (μ moles)/ 10^6 cells
Macrophages + GE-1	-----	29.6 ± 1.71
Macrophages + GE-1	genistein	34.6 ± 1.71
Macrophages + GE-1	tyrphostin	36.3 ± 1.60
Macrophages + AG-83	-----	40.33 ± 2.20
Macrophages + AG-83	genistein	49 ± 1.0
Macrophages + AG-83	tyrphostin	43.66 ± 1.11

[1]Murine peritoneal macrophage monolayers were infected with GE-1 or AG-83 parasites for 2 hr, washed and then incubated with or without PTK antagonists genistein or tyrphostin as described in Materials and Methods.
[2]Nitrite concentrations were determined from the supernatants of 48 hr infected macrophages. Results are mean ± standard deviation of three assays per treatment.

(119, 231, 311, 248). Although, various studies involving protein kinase C, such as chemotactic locomotion in human monocytes (312), c-fos gene expression in murine macrophages (188) and protein phosphorylation in macrophages (313) were reported in Leishmanial infection, signaling events associated with PTKs and PTPases are largely overlooked in this disease. The results from the present study demonstrate that signal transduction events associated with protein tyrosine kinase and phosphatase activities can modulate crucial events during interaction of macrophages with *Leishmania donovani*. The different PTK inhibitors down modulated both virulent and avirulent *Leishmania donovani* promastigote invasion in a dose-dependent manner. In uptake inhibition studies (fig.3A$_1$, 3A$_2$), the PTK inhibitor tyrphostin 25 effectively suppressed *Leishmania donovani* entry at a concentration of 8 μM, while the PTK inhibitor genistein failed to suppress uptake at that level even at 400 μM concentration, probably supporting that these two inhibitors have different mechanisms of action. The inhibitors used in this study presumably down regulated macrophage PTK activity, as treatments were performed prior to infection. Macrophage PTK activity may be induced during interaction of *Leishmania* parasites with macrophages. Interaction of *Leishmania* parasites with macrophages occurs through CR3, CR1 and other integrin receptors of macrophages. Unicellular organisms including *Leishmania* pathogen may interact with integrins directly or by adsorption of ligands such as C3b, C3bi and fibronectin to their surfaces (314). Clustering of integrin receptors of macrophages with Leishmanial ligands may trigger intracellular signaling involving tyrosine phosphorylation like interaction with other mammalian cell membranes (246, 315). However, to understand the role of PTPase in Leishmanial invasion, when we added sodium orthovanadate, an inhibitor of PTPase (316) prior to infection of macrophages, we observed increment in uptake of both virulent and avirulent *Leishmania donovani* promastigotes. Vanadate partially reverted the genistein effects in macrophages when coincubated with both drugs prior to infection (Fig.3C$_1$, 3C$_2$). This observation not only indicates that macrophage tyrosine phosphorylation is involved in the parasite entry but also suggests that vanadate may down-modulate PTPase activity. In contrast, our multiplication study (Fig.3B) showed that PTK inhibitors could not inhibit multiplication of parasites indicating the divergence in signals between entry and replication of these pathogens. Taken together, these data strongly suggest that although virulent and avirulent *Leishmania donovani* parasites induce similar PTK and PTPase signaling pattern for their entry into macrophages, this signal has no relation to the ultimate virulence mechanism associated with intracellular replication of this pathogen.

In the parasite invasion studies, we also demonstrate that parasite uptake by macrophages involves the polymerization of cellular actin (f-actin) and role of this actin polymerization has previously been demonstrated in the entry of bacterial pathogens in many systems (317, 318). A requirement for f-actin formation during parasite internalization was demonstrated by treating monolayers with cytochalasin B, an inhibitor of actin polymerization. A 92% reduction for GE-1, 88% reduction for AG-83 and almost 100% reduction for UR6 in promastigote internalization resulted when macrophages were pretreated with cytochalasin-B, indicating that actin polymerization is the driving force for the uptake of these parasites by macrophages. Binding of the parasite via C3bi or fibronectin to CR3 or other integrin receptors may induce PTK signals, which in turn may send signals to the cytoskeleton and hence the actin polymerization. Intracellular multiplication of various pathogens including *Leishmania* parasites depends upon the level of NO synthase and nitric oxide of host cells (145, 310). In order to correlate the NO_2^- generation with parasite multiplication, NO_2^- production was measured during multiplication of parasites in the presence or absence of PTP inhibitors. Results from NO data (Table-3B) of 48 hr infected macrophages did not differentiate much either with GE-1 or AG-83 strains. In the presence of PTK inhibitors, genistein or tyrphostin, almost similar levels of NO were produced compared to control infected macrophages. This finding not only indicates that PTK inhibitors could interfere much in NO production during multiplication but also suggests that NO may govern in parasite multiplication.

In summary, we propose that invasions of both virulent and avirulent *Leishmania donovani* promastigotes initiate a host cell PTK-dependent response which signals for actin polymerization and thus facilitates phagocytosis. However, this signal has no relation with the ultimate virulence mechanism associated with intracellular replication of this pathogen and intracellular replication well correlated with nitric oxide production. Knowledge of these signaling events will provide a better understanding of basic but largely overlooked aspects of the cell biology of Leishmaniasis.

RECEPTOR-LIGAND INTERACTION BETWEEN *LEISHMANIA DONOVANI* AND MACROPHAGE ALSO INDUCES PROTEIN KINASE C- MEDIATED OXIDATIVE EVENTS DURING ATTACHMENT AND AFTER INTERNALISATION

4

4.1 Introduction

Intramacrophage pathogens like *Leishmania, Mycobacteria, Shigella* and others reside in specific sub-cellular compartments, e.g. a modified phagosome *(Mycobacterium tuberculosis)* (319), the phagolysosome *(Leishmania, Mycobacterium lepraemurium)* (238, 320) or the cytosol (321, 322). Although these pathogens possess different mechanisms for their intracellular compartmentalization, one emerging theme is that, the major effector molecules responsible for the killing of these pathogens are macrophage-derived cytokines or reactive oxygen and nitrogen intermediates. *Leishmania donovani*, the causative agent of visceral Leishmaniasis or Kala-azar, afflicts millions of people worldwide. Before internalization into the host cell, the *Leishmania* pathogen attaches itself onto the host cell surface via complement receptor type 1, type 3, or mannosyl-fucosyl receptor (MFR) of macrophages. Although these pathogens after internalization modulate one or several host functiors, including oxidative metabolism to survive within phagolysosomes, it is still not clearly understood what happens to the oxidative events when the parasite just attaches onto the surface of macrophages i.e., during receptor-ligand interaction. Infection of macrophages with *Leishmania donovani* downregulates one or several protein kinase C (PKC) dependent events in macrophages such as phosphorylation of MARCKS protein (myristoylated alanine-rich C kinase substrate) (313), chemotactic locomotion (312), PMA-stimulated oxygen consumption (323), NADPH-oxidase-mediated superoxide generation (239) and nitrogen dependent mechanisms (324-326) through the secretion of LPG (lipophosphoglycan) or other surface glycoconjugates. Acid phosphatase, another cell surface molecule of *Leishmania*, was found to be associated with decreased amount of superoxide anion production by neutrophils (327). Although the virulency of the parasites may depend upon the expression of these surface molecules, the levels of these surface-expressed molecules on virulent and avirulent *Leishmania donovani* promastigotes and how they differentially regulate in the oxidative metabolism of host cells are still unknown.

In this study, we have examined and compared the PKC-dependent oxidative events of parasite-attached macrophages with macrophages infected either with virulent or avirulent *Leishmania donovani* promastigotes. The findings are discussed in the context of continuation or resolution of infection.

4.2 Materials and Methods

4.2.1 Media and chemicals

RPMI 1640 with L-glutamine, M199, and heat-inactivated fetal bovine serum (FBS) were obtained from GIBCO Laboratories, USA. Cytochalasin D, phorbol-12-myristate-13-acetate (PMA), Staurosporine, tyrphostin AG126, Superoxide dismutase, ferricytochrome C, N-1 -napthylethylene diamine dihydrochloride and sulfanilamide were purchased from Sigma Chemical Co. (St. Louis, MO). All other reagents used were of analytical grade.

4.2.2 Parasites

Leishmania donovani virulent strains GE-1(MHOM/lN/89/GE-1) and AG-83 (MHOM/IN/1983/AG-83) were maintained in female BALB/c mice. Promastigote forms of the parasites were recovered from the spleen of infected mice by adding spleens to culture medium M199 for 5 days at 22°C. *Leishmania donovani* avirulent strain UR6 (MHOM/IN/1978/UR6) was maintained and grown in modified Ray's medium (282) and subcultures were made at 72 hr intervals.

4.2.3 Peritoneal macrophages

Macrophages for infection studies were isolated by peritoneal lavage from female BALB/c mice as described previously (283). Briefly, thioglycollate (TG)-elicited macrophages were isolated from peritoneal cavity and plated in 18 mm cover slips for 2 hr at 37°C. The cells were washed extensively with phosphate buffered saline (PBS) to remove any non-adherent cells. Cells obtained this way were 80-90% viable as tested by trypan blue exclusion test.

4.2.4 Parasite attachment and infection of macrophages

Macrophages (10^7/ml) were treated with the drug cytochalasin D (1.5 μ g/ml) for 1 hr at 37°C before infection and continued to the end of incubation. Macrophages were then challenged with parasites for 2 hr at 37°C at a 10:1 parasite-to-cell ratio. Non-interacted parasites were removed by three washes with warm PBS. In drug-treated macrophages, parasites were found to be attached on macrophage surface, whereas in drug untreated macrophages most of the parasites were found to be internalized. Infection levels were determined by microscopic examination of Giemsa-stained coverslips.

4.2.5 Treatment of macrophages with various kinase inhibitors

Macrophage culture medium was removed from the cells on cover slips and replaced with fresh medium containing protein kinase C inhibitor, staurosporine, 0.1 µM, for 10 mins at 37°C, or protein tyrosine kinase inhibitor, tyrphostin AG126, 20 µM for 30 mins and genistein 10 µM for 30 mins at 37° C.

4.2.6 Oxygen consumption by macrophages

After adherence and treatment with parasites, macrophage cells were scraped by disposable cells scraper and suspended in Krebs-Henseleit buffer (117 mM NaCI/4.7 mM KCI/2.5 mM $CaCl_2$ /1.2mM KH_2 PO_4/1.2 mM $MgSO_4$. $7H_2O$/20 mM Hepes/25 mM $NaHCO_3$, pH7.4). PMA-induced O_2 consumption was measured polargraphically with Clark-type electrodes as described (237).

4.2.7 Measurement of superoxide and nitrite in presence of protein kinase C or protein tyrosine kinase inhibitors

O_2^- was measured by the superoxide dismutase inhibitable reduction of ferricytochrome C (328). Briefly, macrophage cells were incubated in the presence or absence of protein kinase C inhibitor, staurosporine, or protein tyrosine kinase inhibitors, tyrphostin AG 126 or genistein as indicated above. Cells were then washed extensively with PBS and placed in a reaction mixture that contained 80 µM ferricytochrome C, 100 ng/ml PMA in Kreb's Ringer Phosphate glucose with or without 50 µg/ml superoxide dismutase. After 90 min incubation at 37^0C, O_2^- release was determined spectrophotometrically at 550 nm. The production of NO by macrophages was estimated by measuring the accumulation of nitrite, a stable product of NO, by the Greiss reaction. In brief, both normal and infected macrophages were treated with T-cell supernatant (conA-treated) as a source of IFN-γ for first 24 hr and then LPS, 5 µg/ml for another 24 hr. Cell supernatants were then mixed with equal volume of Greiss reagent (0. 5% sulfanilamide and 0.05%-N-1 -napthylethylene diamine hydrochloride in 50% phosphoric acid) and nitrite was measured spectrophotometrically at 550 nm. The concentration of nitrite was determined from a standard curve prepared with sodium nitrite.

4.3 Results

4.3.1 Replication of intracellular *Leishmania donovani* parasites

To study the intracellular replication of parasites, thioglycollate elicited mouse penitoneal macrophages were challenged with the *L.donovani* strains GE-I, AG-83 or UR6 for 2 hr, extracellular parasites were washed off and incubated for various time periods as indicated (Fig.4A). Living promastigotes of GE-I and AG-83 were ingested rapidly compared to UR6 by macrophages over the first 2 hrs after adding the parasites to the cultures. Thereafter, the number of parasites/100 macrophages increased by 3- to

5-fold for GE-I and 2- to 3-fold for AG-83 at 24 hr and 48 hr and began to rise again to give almost 7-fold increase for GE-I and 5-fold for AG-83 by 72 hr. In contrast, for UR6 strains although there was initial increase after 24 hr, the parasites/100 macrophages gradually dropped and by 72 hr the parasite count dropped ~50% indicating that the parasites were probably eliminated by the host cells. Thus, our replication study showed that GE-I was the most virulent among the strains tested.

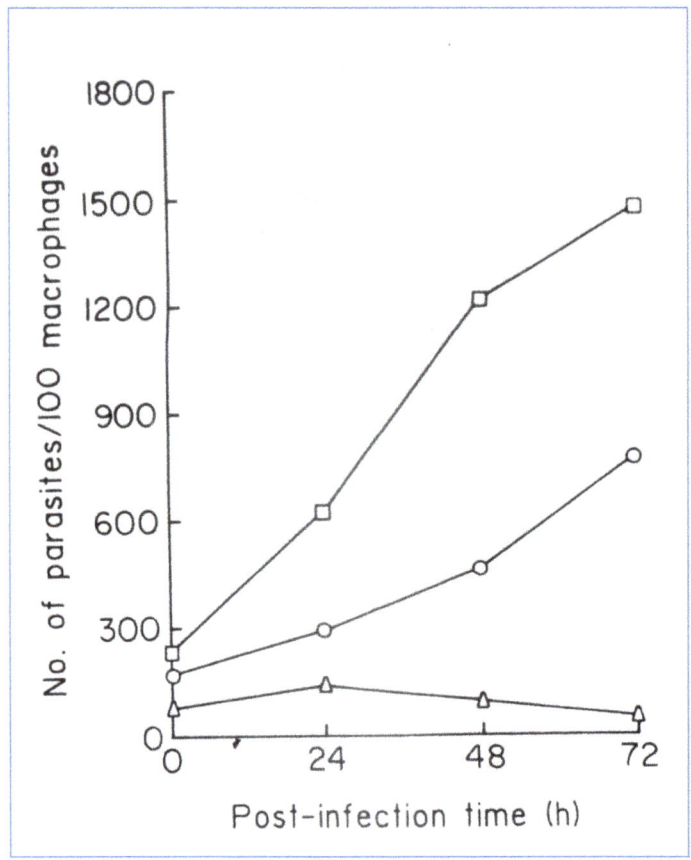

FIG.4A.   Intracellular replication of various strains of *Leishmania donovani* promastigotes. Mouse peritoneal macrophages were exposed to *L. donovani* with either GE-1 strain (□) or AG-83 (o) or UR-6 (Δ) for 2 hr (designated as 0 hr post infection), then cells were washed to remove intracellular parasites and further incubated at 37°C for 24-72 hr in fresh medium for replication. Results are mean of three different experiments performed with duplicate samples.

4.3.2 Oxidative burst activity of *Leishmania donovani* attached or infected macrophages and the role of PKC

Following phagocytosis, because mononuclear phagocytes undergo respiratory burst, we were interested to find out the superoxide generation of macrophages infected with virulent or avirulent *Leishmania donovani* promastigotes. Superoxide production was significantly attenuated in macrophages infected with GE-I and AG-83 strains compared to avirulent strain UR6 (O_2^- with GE-I and AG-83 were 38.33 ± 2.23 and 48± 2.13 n mol/ mg of protein compared to 109.33± 7.9 nmol for UR6 and 81±3.41 nmol for normal) (Fig.4B$_B$). In contrast, direct activation of PKC with PMA, also a known stimulus for O_2^- production, increased O_2^- production, by control cells (Fig.4B$_A$). However, in the presence of cytochalasin-D, when parasites (GE-I and AG-83) were allowed to attach onto macrophage surface, O_2^- generations were increased, and these generations were inhibited significantly in the presence of PKC inhibitor, staurosporine (~46% inhibition) but not in the presence of protein tyrosine kinase inhibitor, tyrphostin AG 126 (Fig.4B$_A$) indicating the role of PKC in the process. Collectively, these results indicated that although parasite attachment induced O_2^- generation, these generations were significantly inhibited during parasite multiplication (~48 hr after infection) and was maximally inhibited for most virulent strain GE-I.

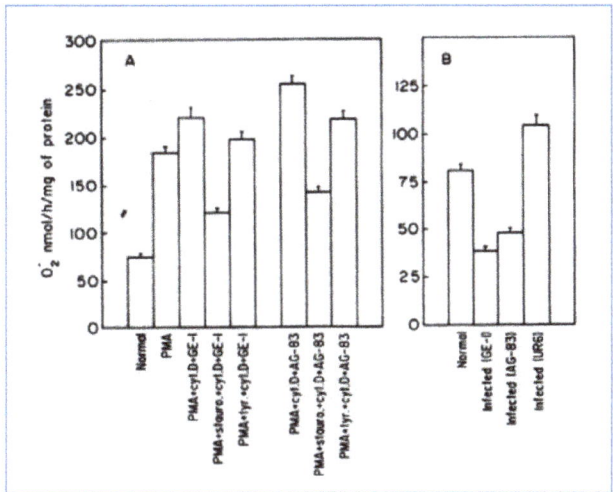

FIG.4B: Superoxide generation of *L. donovani* attached macrophages pretreated with PKC or PTK inhibitors (4B$_A$) and infected macrophages (4B$_B$). MØ monolayers were prepared, preincubated or not with different kinase inhibitors (staurosporine→stauro, tyrphostin→tyr) as described, and then allowed to attach (+Cyt.D) or infect for ~48 hr with different strains of promastigotes. In attachment experiment, MØs were incubated with PMA for 1 hr at 37°C and cultured media were collected for O_2^- assay. Results are mean ± S.D. of three separate experiments.

4.3.3 *Leishmania donovani* attachment does not down regulate oxygen consumption

As known for infected macrophages, inhibition of O_2^- production could be due to defective stimulus-response coupling for activation of the oxidative burst, to scavenging of reactive oxygen intermediates, or to both. To examine this, O_2 consumption was measured for normal, infected and parasite-attached macrophages after PMA treatment. As shown in Fig.4C, compared to normal macrophages, O_2 consumption by macrophages infected with GE-I and AG- 83 was reduced by ~40-50% and for UR6 instead of inhibition there was 4-5% stimulation in O_2 consumption. In contrast, it was found that attachment of different strains of *Leishmania donovani* parasites to macrophages in the presence of cytochalasin D, induced the oxygen consumption substantially (6.69±0.10 nmol/10^6 cells for GE-I attachment compared to 2.93±0.091 for GE-I infection and for AG-83 this was 6.22±0.1 versus 3.54±0.16 and for UR6 it was 7.75±0.15 versus 5.85±0.04).

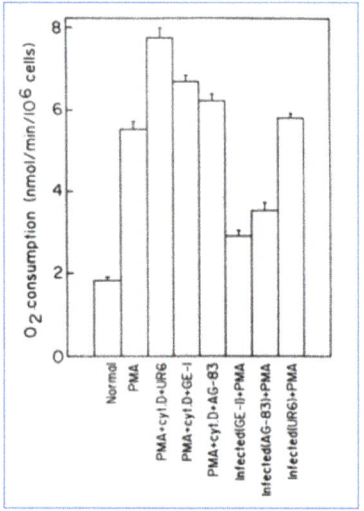

FIG.4C: Oxygen consumption of macrophages during attachment or after infection with virulent versus avirulent *L. donovani* promastigotes. Suspensions of control or *L. donovani* attached (+Cyt.D) or infected (~48 hr) macrophages (10^6/ml) were incubated in the presence or absence of PMA (1 μg/ml for 15 mins.). Data represent mean ± S.D. of results obtained in three independent experiments.

Thus, the above results indicated that, although *Leishmania* attachment to macrophages by all three strains induced almost similar level of O_2 consumption, there was significant reduction in consumption associated with the internalization and multiplication of the parasites and the reduction in consumption was inversely proportional to the virulence of the parasites.

4.3.4 Comparison of NO_2^-- generation during attachment or after infection

It is known that both NO synthase and nitric oxide of macrophages are involved in antibacterial and antiparasitic activity (145, 329). To understand the role of NO in the multiplication of the intracellular parasites, we were interested to estimate the NO_2^-, a stable product of NO. When we compared activated macrophages (crude IFN-γ primed and LPS-treated) with infected macrophages, we found that intracellular GE-1 parasites at 48 hr after infection significantly inhibited the synthesis of NO_2^- (29.66±2.66 μmoles/10^6 cells with GE-I compared to 80.33±4.31 μ moles for control activated macrophage and 70.66±3.10 μmoles for UR6) (Table-4A). Thus the virulent strain GE-I, downregulated the NO_2^- synthesis ~65% whereas the avirulent strain UR6 produced almost similar amount of NO, like control macrophages. On the other hand, attachment of same virulent strain of *Leishmania* (GE-I) to macrophage induced the NO production significantly (110.66±3.10 μmoles/10^6 cells). As, both PKC and PTK play a significant role in NO production, we then examined the effects of these kinase inhibitors on parasite-mediated NO release. As shown in Table 4A, when we used PKC inhibitor, staurosporine, 0.1 µM for 20 mins, NO release was inhibited by ~42%, whereas with the use of PTK inhibitor, genistein and tyrphostin 10 µM for 30 mins, we observed ~60-65% inhibition in NO release. Thus, *Leishmania* attachment induced the release of NO both in PKC and PTK-dependent manner and probably after infection, *Leishmania* parasites, at least virulent strains, downregulate the activity of PKC and PTK to inhibit the production of NO.

4.4 Discussion

The virulence or intracellular survival of a pathogen including *Leishmania* depends upon several factors, involving the surface expression of virulent molecules, their innate resistance to the reactive products of oxidative metabolism, or the failure to induce an oxidative burst that enables them to evade oxygen-dependent killing by their host cells (24, 330). In the present study, before examining how different virulent and avirulent strains of *L.donovani* affect the oxidative events during attachment or after infection of macrophages, we compared their *in vitro* replication pattern. From our *in vitro* replication study, as discussed in detail in the result section, when we compared 72 hr infected macrophages, we found 7-fold increase in parasite burden for GE-I compared to 5-fold increase for AG-83 (Fig.4A). Microscopic examination of Giemsa-stained infected macrophages also suggested us that at 72 hr after infection when multiplication of GE-I and AG-83 parasites were induced, then the counts of UR6 parasites/100 macrophages dropped significantly indicating that they were unable to multiply inside macrophages. Similar type of virulency was also observed from our laboratory in *in vivo* infection of mice (178, 331). Various surface glycoconjugates e.g. LPG, GPI, gp63 and GIPL of *Leishmania* parasites are known to involve in infectivity and intracellular multiplication. Although, nothing much is characterized regarding the fine structure and expression of these surface glycoconjugates on virulent and avirulent *Leishmania donovani* promastigotes, there were many reports on *Leishmania major* and *Leishmania mexicana* (332-335). Recent identification of the defect in lipophosphoglycan biosynthesis in a non-pathogenic strain of *Leishmania major* (336) indicated that similar mechanism might be operative for our least infective strain UR6.

Although infection of macrophages or monocytes with *Leishmania* attenuates several host functions including PMA-stimulated oxygen consumption (323), PKC-mediated protein phosphorylation (313), stimulus response coupling through PKC (237) and Ca^{+2} homeostasis (337). These events were not studied during attachment of parasites to macrophages. However, in the present study, we have observed an induction in cellular activation through superoxide and nitric oxide generation in macrophages during attachment with virulent strains of *Leishmania donovani* promastigotes. Attachment of the parasites to macrophages in the presence of cytochalasin D, an inhibitor of actin polymerization, induced O_2^- generation and O_2 consumption significantly, like PMA, an activator of PKC (Fig.4B$_A$, 4B$_B$, 4C). O_2^- generation was inhibited in the presence of staurosporine, an inhibitor of PKC. However, after infection of macrophages with virulent strain GE-I, significant downregulation in O_2^- generation and O_2 consumption was observed as compared to avirulent strain, UR6. It is known that PKC and its substrate protein phosphorylation might play an important role in O_2^- generation (313, 338). In case of *Leishmania donovani* infected macrophages, defective translocation of PKC (237) and inhibition of phosphorylation of PKC substrate MARCKS protein (313) through leishmanial surface glycoconjugate, LPG was reported. In our previous work (239) with AG-83 but not with GE-I, we showed that PKC-translocation was inhibited in infected macrophages and here we suggest, that could be responsible for observed downregulation of O_2^- generation in macrophages infected with virulent strains. However, during attachment of parasites, we found induction in phosphorylations of at least two macrophage proteins, which might be associated with increased O_2^- generation during attachment.

The production of not only reactive oxygen intermediates, but also the production of nitric oxide from L-arginine by an immune/inflammatory nitric oxide synthase (NOS) by polymorphonuclear leukocytes and macrophages is critical to host defense. Biosynthesis of NO along with O_2^- may lead to the production of several reactive oxynitrogen (RONIs) intermediates, including nitrosonium (NO+) and nitroxyl (NO-) ions, nitrogen dioxide (NO_2), peroxynitrite (ONOO-) and S-nitrosothiols (339), which might be responsible for antibacterial and antiparasitic activity (145, 329). In order to understand the role of NO in intracellular multiplication of different strains of *Leishmania donovani* parasites, in this study, NO_2^- generation was measured after infection of macrophages with virulent or avirulent strains of *Leishmania donovani* promastigotes. NO_2^- generation of infected macrophages was also compared with the generation during attachment of parasites to macrophages. Under attachment condition, in the presence of cytochalasin D, further induction of NO production compared to LPS+IFN-γ activated macrophages was observed (Table-4A). However, this parasite-mediated NO_2^- production was inhibited in the presence of PKC inhibitor, staurosporine and PTK inhibitor, genistein and tyrphostin. During attachment of parasites to macrophages, the receptor-ligand pairing between host and parasite surface might induce both PKC- and PTK-mediated NO signaling pathways and these results are also in agreement with the previous reports that both PKC (340) and PTK (324) are involved in NO-synthase-mediated NO generation from macrophages. In contrast, at 48 hr of post-infection, with virulent strain GE-1 and AG-83, NO production was significantly inhibited compared to UR6. However, generation with UR6 was almost like normal macrophages. Downregulation of NO_2^- generation by GE-1 and AG-83 strains might be due to inhibition of NO-synthase signaling pathway by GIPL or other surface glycoconjugates of intracellular amastigote form of the parasites (341-343).

In conclusion, our findings show that *Leishmania donovani*, both virulent or avirulent strains of parasites, like any other microorganism when attaches to the phagocytes induces PKC-mediated cellular events, however, after infection, only virulent strain significantly downregulates the oxidative events indicating attachment signaling is different from that of infection. Hence, we suggest that impairment of PKC-dependent oxidative events by virulent strains of *Leishmania donovani* may attenuate macrophage activation and contribute to persistence of infection.

TABLE-4A: Effects of PKC and PTK inhibitors on parasite mediated NO release in murine macrophages[1]

Cells	Agents	Nitrite(µ moles)[4] / 10[6] cells
Macrophages (MØs)	LPS	80.33 ± 4.31
MØs + parasite (GE-I)[2]	LPS+Cytochalasin D(Cyt.D)	110.66 ± 3.10
MØs + parasite	LPS+genistein(10 µM)+Cyt.D	45 ± 2.13
MØs + parasite	LPS+tyrphostin(10µM) + Cyt. D	40.66 ± 1.21
MØs + parasite	LPS+staurosporine(0.1µM)+Cyt.D	64 ± 2.41
Infected MØs (GE-I)[3]	LPS	29.66 ± 2.6
Infected MØs (AG-83)	LPS	44.33 ± 2.91
Infected MØs (UR6)	LPS	70.66 ± 3.10

[1] The cells were primed with crude IFN-γ (Con-A treated T-cells supernatant) and then treated with LPS as indicated in materials and methods.

[2] To measure the PKC and PTK-mediated NO release during parasite attachment, macrophages were pre-incubated in the absence or presence of Genistein, Tyrphostin or Staurosporine with the indicated dose, washed, and parasites were added in the presence of cytochalasin-D.

[3] Macrophages infected with different strains of parasites, in absence of cytochalasin-D, when at 48hr after infection, around 8-10 parasites/MØ for GE-1, 3-4 for AG-83 and virtually no UR-6 parasites were detected intracellularly.

[4] These values represent the means ±S.D. of three separate experiments performed with duplicate samples.

ATTACHMENT OF *LEISHMANIA DONOVANI* PROMASTIGOTES INDUCES THE PHOSPHORYLATION AND MYRISTOYLATION OF 29 AND 45-KD MACROPHAGE PROTEINS

5

5.1 Introduction

Leishmania donovani is an intracellular pathogen and the prime cause of the human disease visceral Leishmaniasis or kala-azar. This pathogen infects macrophages of the mammalian systems and enters these cells most efficiently by receptor-mediated endocytosis mechanism, with parasite binding to CR1 and CR3 integrin receptors and mannosyl fucosyl receptor on the surface of the host cell (121, 124, 177).

The process of phagocytosis of a particle or pathogen is initiated when a ligand on the surface of a pathogen or particle becomes engaged with a receptor on the host cell surface. Following binding of ligands, integrin and other receptors on the host cell surface have recently been demonstrated to generate tyrosine or serine and threonine-specific phosporylation signals necessary for the uptake of various particles (344-346). Although, tyrosine-specific phosphorylation signals have previously been demonstrated to play a role in bacterial entry in many systems (119, 293, 347-349), the role of protein kinase C (PKC)-specific phosphorylation in the promotion of bacteria as well as Leishmanial entry has not been established. However, PKC-specific phosphorylation has been reported in zymosan phagocytosis by macrophages (350) and Fc receptor-mediated phagocytosis by monocytes (351). Likewise protein phosphorylation, role of myristoylations of several PKC-substrate proteins in Leishmanial entry has also not been previously studied. However, role of MARCKS (myristoylated alanine rich C kinase substrate) and macMARCKS, a novel member of the MARCKS family has been demonstrated in the uptake of different particles (350, 352).

In the present study, we therefore have investigated protein phosphorylation and myristoylation pattern of macrophages during attachment with *L. donovani* promastigotes. We demonstrated that PKC-mediated specific proteins were phosphorylated with exogenous orthophosphate and acylated with exogenous myristic acid when macrophages were stimulated with attachment of *L. donovani*. Phosphorylation and myristoylation of these specific proteins were also compared with the macrophages after established infection. The role of these specific proteins in the context of recognition, uptake and intracellular survival of *L. donovani* promastigotes in permissive macrophages are discussed.

5.2 Materials and Methods

5.2.1 Media and Chemicals

Medium 199, penicillin, streptomycin, gentamycin were from Gibco Laboratories, Grand Island, NY, USA. RPMI-1640, Fetal bovine serum (FBS) (heat inactivated) were from Difco, USA. Staurosporine, leupeptin, aprotinin, pepstatin, phenyl methyl sulfonyl fluoride (PMSF), PMA, *E. coli* LPS, cytochalasin-D, NaF, NaH_2PO4, $NaHPO_4$, sodium pyrophosphate, EDTA, EGTA, Vanadate, ATP were from Sigma. 9, 10(n)– ^{3}[H]–myristic acid is from Amersham-pharmacia Biotech, ^{32}[P]-orthophosphate from BARC, India and all other reagents used were of analytical grade.

5.2.2 Parasites

L. donovani virulent strains AG83 (MHOM/IN/1983/AG83) and GE-1(MHOM/IN/89/GE-1) strains were maintained in female BALB/c mice as described previously (178). Parasites were recovered from the spleen of infected mice by adding spleens to culture medium M199 supplemented with 20% FBS, 100 µg/ml penicillin and 100 µg/ml streptomycin. The cultures were kept for 5 days at 22°C to obtain promastigotes, which were then washed and used for infection of macrophages. Bacterial strains, *E. coli* DH-5α and *Shigella flexneri* were gifts from Dr. Rupak Bhadra of our Infectious Disease Group, IICB.

5.2.3 Peritoneal macrophages

Macrophages were isolated as previously described (283, 239). Briefly, thioglycollate (TG)-elicited macrophages were isolated by peritoneal lavage from male BALB/c mice. Four days after TG-injection, cells were isolated from the peritoneal cavity, by washing with 3-4 ml of RPMI-1640 medium supplemented with 25 mM HEPES, 100 µg/ml streptomycin, 100 µg/ml penicillin and 20% of FBS. Cells were then plated onto 22 mm coverslips and allowed to adhere at 37°C for 2 hrs. Nonadherent cells were washed out by extensive washing with PBS. Cells obtained this way were 80-90% viable as tested by trypan blue exclusion method.

5.2.4 Attachment or infection of macrophages with parasites

Macrophages (10^7/ml) were treated with the drug cytochalasin D (1.5 µg/ml) for 1 hr at 37°C before infection and continued to the end of incubation with parasites. *L. donovani* promastigotes or bacterial strains *E. coli* or *Shigella flexneri* were then added to macrophage monolayers at a 10:1 parasite-to-cell ratio and kept at 37°C for 1-2 hrs. For established infection, cells were incubated in the absence of the drug. Non-interacted parasites were removed by three washes with warm PBS. For intracellular replication, macrophage cells were kept in culture for additional 24-72 hrs. Attachment or infection levels were determined by microscopic examination of Giemsa-stained cells.

5.2.5 Protein phosphorylation in parasite-interacted macrophages

Phosphorylation of macrophage proteins in response to interaction with parasite was detected as previously described (353) with minor modifications. In brief, macrophage monolayers were washed four times with phosphate-free DMEM or loading buffer (LB) [10mM Hepes, 2.7 mM KCl, 138mM NaCl, 7.5 mM D-glucose] and then incubated for 4 hrs at 37°C in this medium containing 250-300 µci of [^{32}P] orthophosphoric acid per ml. At the end of this incubation, macrophages were treated with *L. donovani* promastigotes or different bacterial species for 30 min-1 hour in the presence of cytochalasin D as indicated in the legend of the Figs. For phosphorylation in established infection, infected macrophage cultures were incubated at 37°C in 5% CO_2 for 24hr-72hr and then labelled with [^{32}P] orthophosphoric acid. After incubation, the macrophage monolayers were washed with cold PBS and then scraped in homogenizing buffer (HB) (0.25M sucrose, 20 mM Hepes, 0.5 mM EGTA, pH 7.0), containing protease inhibitors (2 mM leupeptin, 0.5 mM PMSF, 10µg/ml pepstatin, 10µg/ml aprotinin) and phosphatase inhibitors (10 mM NaF, 5 mM EDTA, 1 mM ATP, 10 mM NaH_2PO_4, 10 mM Na_2HPO_4, 5mM disodium pyrophosphate). The cells were then pelleted and solubilized in sodiumdodecyl sulphate-polyacrylamide gel electrophoresis (SDS-PAGE) (368) sample buffer and then incubated at 95°C for 10 min. Samples (~8 x 10^4 cpm) were electrophoresed in 8 or 10% polyacrylamide gels containing SDS and subsequently stained with coomassie brilliant blue and destained. Dried gels were exposed to Kodak X-OMAT film with intensifying screens to detect changes in the [^{32}P] -labelling of the various proteins.

5.2.6 Myristoylation of macrophage proteins

Myristoylation of proteins was detected according to the method of Aderem et.al (354). In short, macrophages cultured at a density of 3-5 x 10^6 cells per plate were washed 3-4 times with PBS and incubated for the indicated times in 1 ml of DMEM containing 25-30 µci [3$_H$] myristic acid (20 - 40 ci/mmol, 1 ci = 37GBq)- defatted BSA complex per ml for 2h at 37°C. [3$_H$] myristic acid defatted BSA complex was first made by adding 1 mg/ml of defatted BSA in DMEM minus FBS, shaken, [3$_H$]-myristic acid added and required volume made up with DMEM plus FBS. In one preparation, macrophages were preincubated with ConA-stimulated T-cell supernatant for 24hr and then treated with [3$_H$]-myristic acid. ConA-stimulated T-cell supernatant was used as a source of crude IFN-γ. Specified stimuli as indicated in the Fig. legends of *L. donovani* promastigotes AG-83 or GE-I was then added and incubated for one hour at 37°C in the presence of cytochalasin D. At the end of the specified incubation time, the cells were washed three times with PBS and scraped in homogenizing buffer containing protease inhibitors plus 1 mM diisopropyl fluorophosphate and 15 mM EDTA. Cells were then pelleted, solubilized and the protein content was determined according to the method of Lowry et al (286). Samples containing equivalent amounts of protein were subjected to SDS-PAGE on 8-10% acrylamide gel according to Laemmli (355). Proteins were fixed, stained and prepared for fluorography by treatment with PPO POPOP (356).

5.3 Results

5.3.1 Protein phosphorylation of macrophages after *L.donovani* attachment

Incubation of mouse macrophage monolayers for 1-2 hr with a virulent strain GE-I of *L. donovani* in the presence of cytochalasin D (Fig.5A1), triggered phosphorylation of multiple proteins, including 29-, 45-, 67- and 95-kDa proteins (Fig.5A$_2$, 5A$_3$, lane-4). However, 29- and 45 kDa bands were obtained from phosphorylation of most prominent proteins. Phosphorylation profiles were slightly better in DMEM than in loading buffer. Addition of PMA, an activator of PKC further induced the phosphorylation of these proteins. Qualitative scanning (pixel intensity, Fig.5A$_3$) of the autoradiograph and the summary of the scan (Table-5A) demonstrated that attachment of cells with *L. donovani* parasites induced the phosphorylation of 29- and 45-kDa proteins significantly. Scanning data demonstrated that the pixel intensity of 29-kDa protein in PMA-induced *L. donovani* attached macrophages was 119±7.12 (n=4) (in DMEM) and 85±3.51 (in loading buffer) compared to 50.25±3.92 (in OMEM) in normal macrophages. Similarly, pixel intensity for 45-kDa protein was 58.5±3.16 compared to not detectable in normal macrophages. Thus attachment of *L. donovani* GE-I strain in unstimulated or PMA-stimulated macrophage cells triggered selectively the phosphorylation of 29- and 45-kDa proteins.

5.3.2 Attachment versus established infection: comparison of protein phosphorylation

We next tried to examine whether parasite attachment signal in phosphorylation differs with macrophages after established infection. In order to develop established infection, macrophages were infected with *L. donovani* virulent strain GE-I for approximately 48-72 hr, and the level of infection is shown in (Fig.5B$_1$). Infected macrophages were then labelled with [^{32}P]-orthophosphate and phosphorylation was compared with cytochalasin D treated *L. donovani* attached macrophages (Fig-5B$_2$). Infection with the virulent strain GE-I for 48 hr at an infectivity ratio of 10 parasites per macrophage significantly downregulated the phosphorylations of 29- and 45- kDa proteins. Although phosphorylations of both 29- and 45-kDa proteins were significantly downregulated in infected macrophages, 45 kDa protein was not at all visible in 48 hr infected macrophages. Comparison of scanning (Fig. 5A$_3$, 5B$_3$, Table 5B) of attachment versus

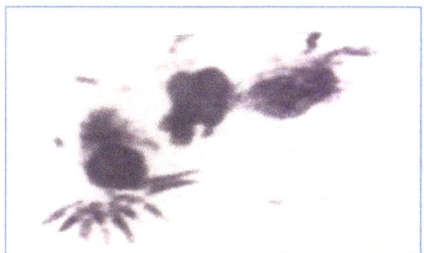

Fig. 5A₁

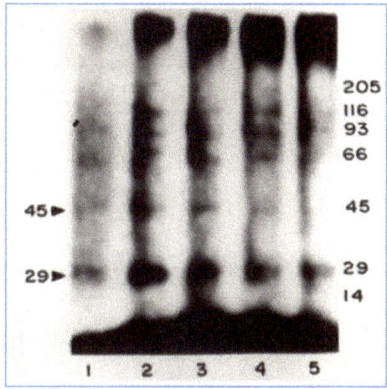

Fig. 5A₂

FIG. 5A1, 5A2: *Leishmania donovani* attachment induced phosphorylation of mouse macrophage proteins. (5A₁) Attachment of *L. donovani* virulent strains, GE-I, with macrophages in presence of cytochalasin D. Cytochalasin D treatment (1.5 µg/ml) was done hr before infection and continued to the end of incubation. Cells were fixed; Giemsa stained and photographed under 100x oil immersion. The picture was then scanned through Adobe photoshop→6 versions, 400 dpi resolution via Hewlett Packard Scanjet 5300 C Scanner.
(5A₂) Shown protein phosphorylation in macrophages at attachment with *L. donovani* promastigote. Macrophage monolayers either in DMEM or in loading buffer (see, "Materials and Methods) were labelled with 250-300 µci ³²Pi/ml for 2-3 hr at 37°C. Cells were then incubated with promastigotes of cytochalasin D and then stimulated with or without PMA. The cells were solubilized in Laemmli buffer and subjected to SDS-PAGE followed by autoradiography. Lane 1, normal macrophage cells; lane 2, *L. donovani* attached PMA-stimulated cells in DMEM; lane 3, same as lane 2 but in loading buffer; lane 4, *L. donovani* attached but without PMA stimulated cells in DMEM; lane 5, same as lane 4 but in loading buffer.

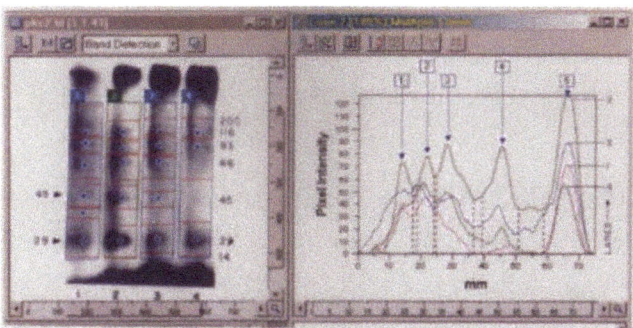

FIG. 5A3: Qualitative scanning of the autoradiograph (5A₂), analysed by Image Master Elite. Arrows indicates the lanes as in (5A₂) and molecular sizes of the proteins. (6) Indicates 29 kD proteins (5), 45 kD(4)67 kd, (3)95 kD, (2) 116 kD and (1) 205 kD proteins for lane 2 and similarly for other lanes.

TABLE - 5A: (Summary of the Scan-5A3)

Lane	Cells+ treatment	Band (kD)	Pixel intensity ± S.D*
01	MØ (normal)	29	50.25 ± 3.92
		45	--
02	MØ+PMA+Cyto-D+ *L.donovani* (GE-I) (DMEM medium)	29	119 ± 7.12
		45	58.5 ± 3.16
03	MØ + PMA + Cyto - D+ *L.donovani* (GE-I) (Loading buffer)	29	85 ± 3.51
		45	34.5 ± 2.26
04	MØ + Cyto-D + *L.donovani* (GE-I) (DMEM medium)	29	85.25 ±2.62
		45	36.25 ± 2.58
05	MØ + Cyto-D+ *L.donovani* (GE-I) (Loading buffer)	29	70.87 ± 4.41
		45	29.75 ± 2.70

* Pixel intensity values are mean of four different autoradiographs ± S.D.
MØ-Macrophage; CytoD-Cytochalasin D

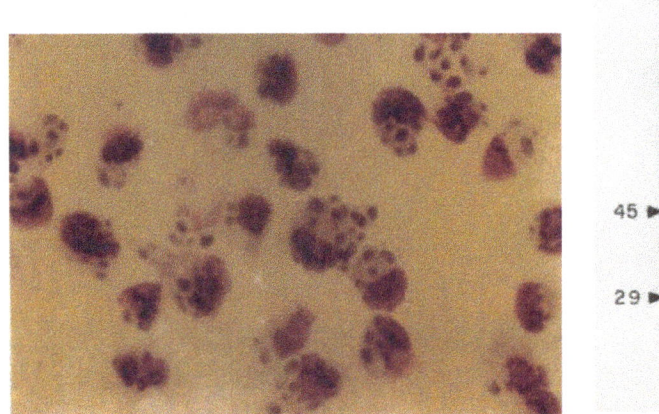

Fig.5B₁

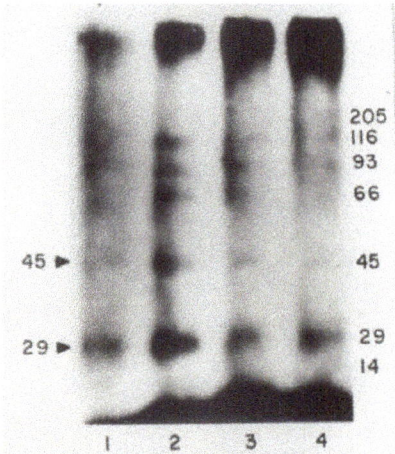

Fig.5B₂

FIG. 5B1, 5B2: Protein phosphorylation in macrophages attached or infected with a virulent strain (GE-I) of *L. donovani* (5B₁). Infected macrophages showing intracellular *L. donovani* amastigotes after 48 hr of infection. Macrophages were incubated with the parasites for 2 hr in absence of cytochalasin D, washed and left for 48 hr in CO_2 incubator for replication, washed, stained and scanned as described in Fig.5A₁, 5B₂. Autoradiograph of the experiment performed with infected macrophage versus *L. donovani* attached macrophage. 48 hr infected macrophages were labelled with ^{32}P and cellular phosphoproteins were analysed by SDS-PAGE and compared with phosphoproteins of macrophages attached with *L. donovani* promastigotes. [32]P labelling for attachment experiment was done as described in Fig. 5A₂ Lane 1, normal macrophage cells; lane 2, *L. donovani* -attached macrophages; lane 3, 24hr infected macrophages; lane 4, 48hr infected macrophages.

established infection indicated that pixel intensities for 45 kDa proteins were 85.93 for attachment and 41.25 and not detected respectively for 24 hr and 48 hr infection. Similarly, for 29-kDa protein the pixel intensities were 126.67 for attachment compared to 52.75 for 24 hr infection and 39.87 for 48 hr infection. These results therefore suggest that although the phosphorylation is induced during the attachment of *L. donovani* promastigotes to the surface of the macrophage, the phosphorylation of these proteins drastically reduced during the growth of the parasites inside macrophages.

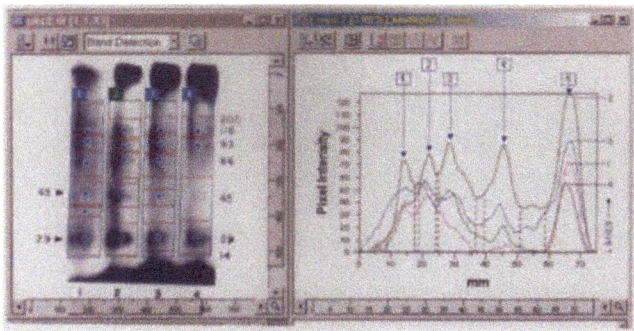

FIG.5B3: Scanning of the autoradiograph, 5B₂. Lanes and molecular sizes of the proteins are marked by arrows. (5) indicates 29 kDprotein; (4) 45kD, (3) 67 kD, (2) 95 kD and (1) for 116 kD protein and similarly for other lanes.

TABLE – 5B: (Summary of the Scan-5E2)

Lane	Cells+ treatment	Band (kD)	Pixel intensity ± S.D*
01	MØ + Cyto-D + L.*donovani*(GE-I)	29 45	30.25 ± 0.87 22.6± 1.79
02	MØ + ConA(T cell supernatant) +Cyto-D+L.*donovani* (GE-I)	29 45	52.75 ± 0.91 39.87 ± 2.07
03	MØ + Cyto D+ L.*donovani* (GE-I)	29 45	126.67 ± 1.78 85.93
04	MØ + LPS+CytoD+L.*donovani* (GE-I)	29 45	41.25 ± 1.66 ---
05	MØ (Normal)	29 45	20.00 ± 1.09 16.00 ± 1.69

Pixel intensity values are mean of four different autoradiographs ± S.D.
Cyto D-Cytochalasin D

5.3.3 Inhibitor of protein kinase C blocks protein phosphorylation

In our previous experiments, we have observed further induction in phosphorylations during addition of PMA, an activator of PKC in *L. donovani* attached macrophages. To confirm further the role of PKC in the phosphorylation process, we did phosphorylation reaction in the presence of staurosporine, an inhibitor of PKC. Macrophage cells were preincubated with staurosporine (1 µM) for 15-30 min prior to further processing for phosphorylation reactions. Treatment of cells with staurosporine resulted in decreased expression of 29- and 45-kDa protein (Fig. 5C₁, lane-3). The actual decrease in the intensity of these bands was found from the scanning of the autoradiograph (Fig.5C₂). Pixel intensity values of the 45-KDa band for *L. donovani* attached macrophages was 66.78 compared to 20.05 in staurosporine-treated macrophages, and for 29-kDa band it was 110.52 in parasite-attached macrophages compared to 64.52 in staurosporine-treated macrophages indicating the role of PKC in the phosphorylation reaction.

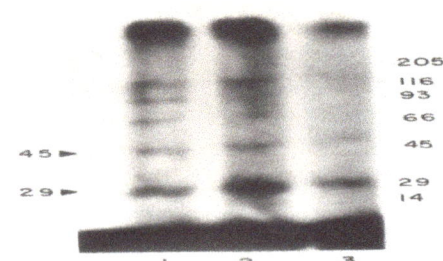

Fig. 5C₁

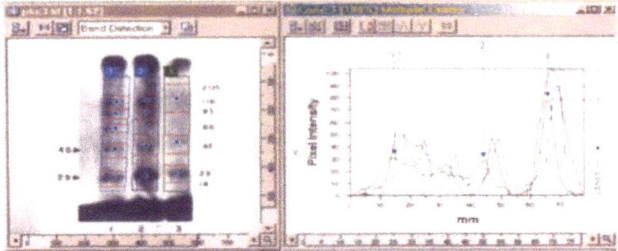

Fig. 5C₂

FIG. 5C1, 5C2:   Protein phosphorylation in macrophages pre-treated with staurosporine, an inhibitor of protein kinase C. (5C₁) Autoradiograph of the staurosporine treated phosphorylation experiment. Macrophage monolayers were pre-treated with or without staurosporine as described in Materials and Methods. Parasites were added in the presence or absence of cytochalasin D. Cells were solubilized, subjected to electrophoresis and autoradiography. Lane 1, normal macrophages; lane 2, *L. donovani* attached, PMA-stimulated macrophage cells; lane-3, staurosporine treated, **L. donovani** attached macrophages. 5C₂ scanning of the autoradiograph, 5C₁ Lanes and molecular sizes of the proteins scanned are shown by arrows. (1) indicates 116 kD protein; (2) 93 kD, (3) 66 kD, (4) 45 kD and (5) for 29 kD proteins and similarly for other lanes.

5.3.4 Analysis of parasite-specific induction of phosphoproteins

We next tested whether the induction in protein phosphorylation was *L. donovani* specific or the exposure of macrophages to other pathogens would also induce the observed protein phosphorylations. For this, [^{32}P]- orthophosphate labelled macrophages were incubated with either *L. donovani* promastigotes or *E. coli* or *Shigella flexneri* in the presence or absence of cytochalasin D. All these species successfully internalises into macrophages (Fig.5D$_{1-3}$) (357, 358). Studies with *E.coli* or *Shigella flexneri*, using the same conditions as those with *L. donovani* were performed for comparative purposes. Figs.5D$_4$ and 5D$_5$ are representatives of autoradiographic and scanning data. These data show that although *E.coli* internationalization produces slightly more intense bands for 29- and 45-kDa proteins (Fig.5D$_4$, lane-6), attachment of macrophages with these bacteria was ineffective at inducing the phosphorylation of 29- and 45-kDa proteins.

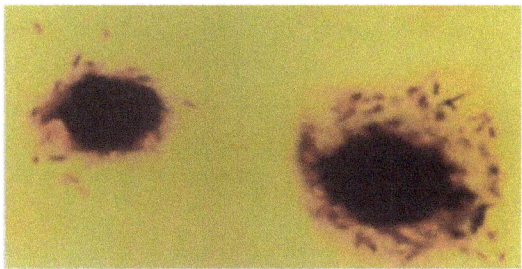

Fig.5D₁

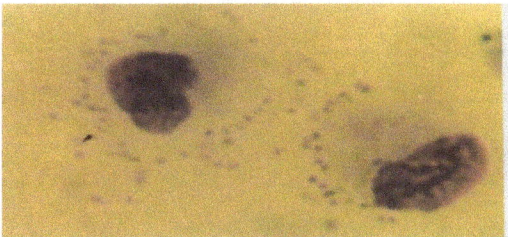

Fig.5D₂

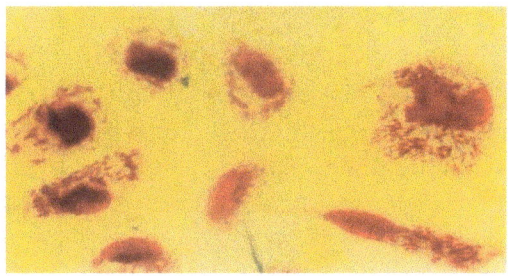

Fig.5D₃

FIG. 5D1-3:   Shown attachment of ***E. coli*** (5D₁), *Shigella flexneri* (5D₂) and infection of ***E.coli*** (5D₃) with macrophages. Macrophages were incubated with *E.coli, Shigella flexneri* in the presence or absence of cytochalasin D, washed, fixed and scanned as in Fig. 5A₁.

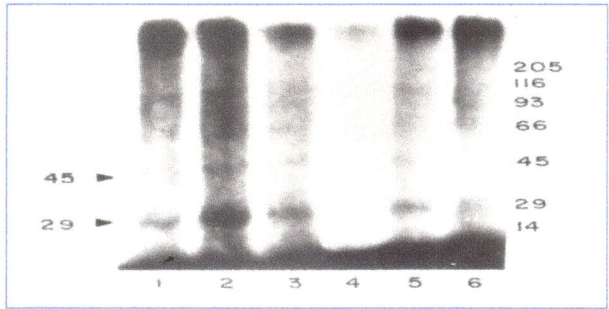

FIG. 5D4:   Autoradiograph of the phosphorylation experiment performed with macrophages attached or infected with different pathogens. Lane 1, normal macrophages; lane 2, *L.donovani* - attached macrophages, lane 3, *L. donovani,* 2hr infected macrophages; lane 4, *E.coli* attached macrophages; lane 5, *Shigella flexneri* attached macrophages; lane 6; *E.coli,* 1 hr infected macrophages.

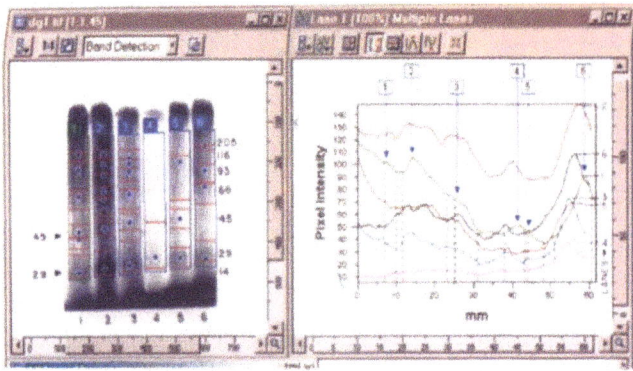

FIG. 5D5: Scanning of the autoradiograph, 5D₄. Lanes and molecular sizes of the proteins scanned are shown by arrows (1) indicates 205 kD protein, (2) 116 kD, (3)93 kD, (4) 67 kD (5) 45 kD and (6) for 29 kD protein and similarly for other lanes.

5.3.5 Attachment of *L. donovani* also induces myristoylation of macrophage PKC-specific proteins

As, MARCKS (myristoylated alanine rich C kinase substrate), mac-MARCKS and other related proteins and their expressions in macrophages play an important role in the uptake of various particles [350, 352, 364], we thought it would be worthwhile to study whether *L. donovani* attachment could affect in the myristoylation of macrophage proteins. To study this, macrophages were cultured for 2 hr with [3_H]-myristic acid-defatted BSA complex and then incubated with or without *L. donovani* promastigotes and cytochalasin D. Autoradiography (Fig.5E$_1$) of normal macrophages (lane 5 of 5E$_1$) shows a basal myristoylation of several proteins particularly 18-, 50- and 90- kDa species. Attachment of *L. donovani*, GE-I (Fig.5E$_1$, lane 1,3 and Table5B) or AG-83 strain (Fig.5F$_1$), clearly induced specific myristoylation of a 29-kDa species and likely to be a doublet of 42-45 kDa, but did not affect the extent of myristoylation of the 14 or 18-kDa proteins compared to that seen in untreated cells. Preincubation of macrophage cells with conA-stimulated T-cell supernatant or addition of LPS further induced those specific bands as demonstrated by autoradiograph, scan (Fig.5E$_1$, lane-2, 4 and 5E$_2$) and Table 5$_B$. Gel scan values indicated that pixel intensities for 29-kDa protein in T-cell sup. stimulated *L.donovani* attached macrophages was 52.75±0.91 (n=4) compared to 20±1.09 in normal macrophages and for 42-45 kDa protein, it was 41.25±2.07 for *L.donovani* attached macrophages compared to 16±1.69 in untreated macrophages. Similarly, for LPS treated *L. donovani* attached macrophages, pixel intensity value for 29-kDa protein was 46.75±1.66 and for 42-45 kDa species it was 39.87 ± 1.76. Although, during protein phosphorylation, we have observed the induction in PKC-mediated phosphorylations of 29- and 45-kDa proteins and induced myristoylated proteins but it is difficult to tell whether those were PKC-specific proteins or not. Further studies are needed for the confirmation. These results collectively suggest that both LPS and T-cell supernatant helped to trigger macrophage protein myristoylations and *L.donovani* attachment further induced the process.

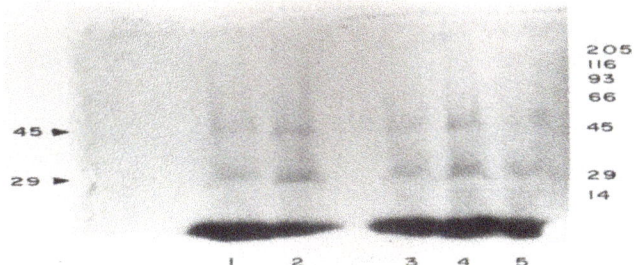

Fig.5E₁

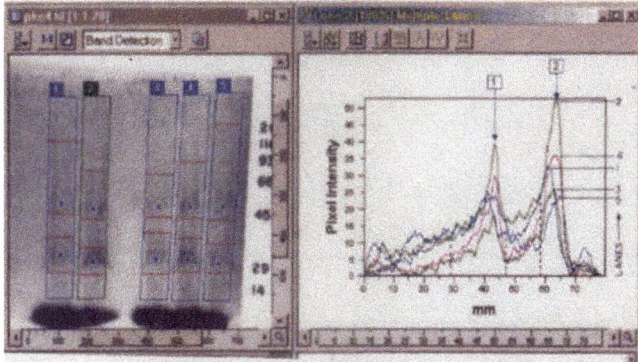

Fig.5E₂

FIG.5E1,5E2:   *Leishmania donovani* attached — dependent incorporation of [3$_H$] myristic acid into macrophage proteins (5E$_1$) Fluorographic of the gel performed after myristoylation of macrophage proteins in relation with *L. donovani*, GE-I attachment. Thioglycollate elicited peritoneal macrophages were incubated in 1 ml of DMEM containing 25-30 µci of [3$_H$] myristic acid-defatted BSA complex and the following stimuli: lane 1 and 3 cytochalasin D + *L. donovani*, GE-I strain: lane 2, T-cell supernatant + cytochalasin D+ *L. donovani*, Lane 4, LPS + cytochalasin D + *L. donovani*; lane 5, no stimulus. After incubation, cells were scraped into HB buffer, pelleted, and analysed by SDS-PAGE, followed by fluorography (PPO-POPOP method). The fluorograph shown was exposed for 4 weeks. (5E$_2$). Scanning of the fluorograph, 5E$_1$ Lanes and molecular sizes of the proteins are marked by arrows. (1) indicates 42-45 kD protein, and (2), 29 kD protein and similarly for other lanes.

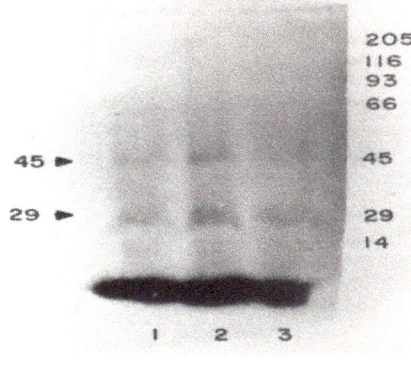

Fig.5F₁

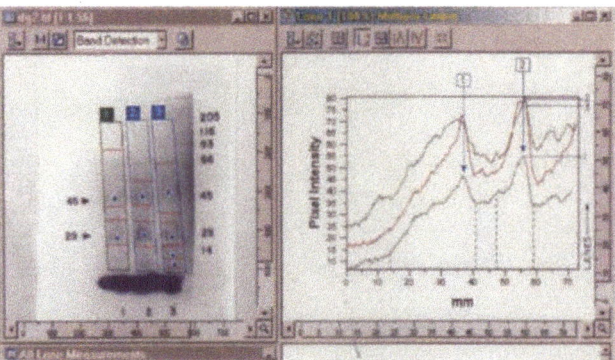

Fig.5F₂

FIG.5F1, 5F2: *Leishmania donovani,* AG-83 strain-dependent myristoylation of macrophage proteins. (5F₁) Fluorograph of the myristoylation experiment performed in the presence of *L.donovani* AG-83 strain. Thioglycollate elicited peritoneal macrophages were incubated as described for Fig.5F with [3$_H$] myristic acid defatted BSA complex and the following stimuli: lane 1, cytochalasin D + *L.donovani,* AG-83 strain; lane 2, LPS + Cytochalasin D + *L.donovani,* AG-83 strain; lane 3, no stimulus. After incubation, the cells were processed as for 5F₁. The fluorograph was exposed for ~25 days. (5F₂), Scanning of the fluorograph, 6A. Lanes and molecular sizes of the proteins are marked by arrows. (1) indicates ~42-45 kD protein; (2) 29 kD protein and similarly for other lane.

5.4 Discussion

Protein phosphorylation and dephosphorylation regulate various functions of host cells in response to different stimulus such as bacterial lipopolysaccharides to bacterial pathogens. Binding of the stimulus (ligand) to the surface receptor of various kinds of immune cells including macrophages has been demonstrated to induce phosphorylations of certain cellular proteins (201, 359). Although there were some preliminary works including a report indicating that attachment of a virulent bacterial pathogen *Legionella pneumophilla* induced phosphorylation of a 76-kDa protein in macrophages, to our knowledge, however, similar observations have not been reported for macrophages attached with *Leishmania* parasites. In this study, we have shown that *L. donovani* attachment induces the phosphorylation and myristoylation of at least four proteins including 29- and 45-kDa proteins in primary macrophage cultures.

L. donovani uses several macrophage surface receptors including MFR, receptor for advanced glycosylation end products and integrin receptors for their attachment and entry (121, 124, 177, 360). Interaction with integrin receptors has recently been demonstrated to send signals through both PKC- and PTK-mediated phosphorylated proteins for bacterial entry in many systems (344-346, 361). Our study also shows that attachment of a virulent strain GE-I of *L.donovani* in the presence of cytochalasin D induces phosphorylation of at least two proteins 29- and 45-kDa of macrophages as confirmed by Fig.5A₂ and its corresponding scanning (Fig.5A₃). Addition of PMA, an activator of PKC further induced the phosphorylation of these proteins (Fig.5A₂) and staurosporine, an inhibitor of PKC blocked the phosphorylation (Fig. 5C₁) of the proteins, confirming the involvement of PKC in the process. Although tyrosine-specific phosphorylation signals have previously been demonstrated in bacterial entry in many systems (344-346), recent reports on various particles (350, 351) and few pathogens including *E.coli* invasion in HEp-2 cells (362) and *Legionella pneumophilla* entry into human monocytes (23) are shown to be PKC-mediated. We also suggest here that interaction of *L.donovani* promastigote with probably integrin receptors activated PKC and in turn induced the phosphorylation of 29- and 45-kDa proteins. This is further supported by the previous report (363) that *Leishmania* attachment is associated with increased intracellular Ca^{+2} influx and DAG, which subsequently may activate PKC, and also in agreement with our previous observation that *L.donovani* attachment induces PKC-mediated oxidative events. In contrast, other intramacrophage pathogens such as *Shigella flexneri* and *E.coli* could not induce the PKC-specific phosphorylation (Fig.5D$_4$) as those observed with *L.donovani* attachment indicating that observed phosphorylations of 29- and 45-kDa proteins might be selectively associated with the attachment by a virulent strain of *L.donovani*. However, after established infection, the expression of these proteins was significantly downregulated as reported by us (Fig. 5B$_2$) and others (237, 313) suggesting that PKC-mediated protein phosphorylation was not required for parasite replication once they entered the host cell.

PKC-specific various myristoylated substrate proteins like MARCKS, macMARCKS and MARCKS related protein (MRP) also are known to be involved in various macrophage functions including pseudopod extension, spreading, phagocytosis and uptake of different particles (350, 352, 199, 364). Membrane anchoring of these proteins after myristoylation might assist the cells to perform above functions. In order to study the involvement of macrophage myristoylated proteins in *Leishmania* phagocytosis, we examined myristoylation of macrophage proteins during attachment with *L.donovani* promastigotes. Surprisingly, we observed the induction in myristoylation of at least two proteins at the region of 29- and 42-45 kDa (Fig. 5E$_1$). Although a recent report (365) indicated that 42 kDa protein is mac-MARCKS, further studies are needed to confirm whether the induced proteins are PKC substrate proteins or not. Preincubation of the cells with T-cell supernatant (IFN-γ source) or LPS and post-treatment with *L.donovani* in the presence of cytochalasin D significantly induced the expression of these proteins (Fig.5E$_1$). It is known that LPS, IFN-γ are important regulatory molecules for macrophage activation and myristoylation of various macrophage proteins (354, 366) might participate as intermediate steps of this activation process. We therefore suggest that attachment of *L.donovani* to LPS or IFN-γ treated cells might further induce the activation process via myristoylations of these proteins and subsequently this could induce the phagocytosis and uptake of these pathogens. Furthermore, in addition to 42-kDa mac-MARCKS protein there could be several kinases including protein kinase C (367) that might get translocated to plasma membrane upon myristoylation during attachment with parasites. The translocated kinases could then phosphorylate appropriate substrate proteins for parasite uptake.

In conclusion, the data obtained in this study suggested that the process of *L.donovani* attachment generated a variety of PKC-mediated inducive molecular signalling within the macrophages and these events significantly downregulated after established infection. Indeed, we found the inductions in 29- and 45-kDa phosphorylated proteins and myristoylations also at the same region but not in cells attached to *E.coli* or *Shigella flexneri*. These results indicated that the phosphorylations and myristoylations of these proteins might be a unique event associated with the recognition and uptake of *L.donovani* pathogens by macrophages and phosphorylations of these proteins were not required for intracellular replication of these pathogens.

INVOLVEMENT OF MACROPHAGE PROTEIN KINASE C DURING INTRACELLULAR REPLICATION OF *LEISHMANIA DONOVANI*

6

6.1 Introduction

Leishmania, the causative agent of Leishmaniasis, resides and proliferates within the hostile environment of phagolysosomes (368) of host macrophages. One of the primary microbicidal activities of phagolysosomes is the oxidative burst, an event that is very critical to host defense. The parasite may alter this pathway to survive. Activation of the oxidative burst and generation of superoxide (O_2^-) in phagocytes are directly dependent on the protein kinase C (PKC) system (369). Although LPG, a cell-surface molecule of *Leishmania donovani*, inhibited PKC-dependent events such as chemotactic locomotion in human monocytes (312), c-fos gene expression in murine macrophages (188) and attenuated PMA-stimulated oxygen consumption (323), nothing is known about the kinetics of activation and desensitisation of PKC in macrophages, particularly their role in alteration of membrane fluidity and their consequences on uptake and further infection.

PKC is a well-characterized example of calcium and phospholipid-dependent cellular kinases, which play a pivotal role in the regulation of a variety of cell functions (370). In cells, these kinases are translocated and activated in response to stimulation by hormones or phorbol esters (363). PMA, a well-known phorbol ester, has been shown to activate (371) and deplete (372) PKC from cells depending upon the incubation period. Stimulation of cells with PMA increases intracellular concentrations of diacylglycerol, which induces translocation of PKC from cytosol to the plasma membrane of the cells. Activation of PKC results in phosphorylation of several proteins in different cell systems including phagocytes, which in turn activates NADPH oxidase (234). The functional end points of this signal transduction cascade in phagocytic cells are superoxide generation (235).

Because the initial attachment of *Leishmania* promastigotes to macrophages is receptor-mediated, the expression of the receptor may play a vital role in the interaction of parasites with macrophages. In erythrocytes and macrophages, the expression of receptors has been shown to be significantly altered by changes in the membrane microviscosity (86,

87). As lipid-protein association is one of the major parameters which controls membrane microviscosity, it is presumed that depletion of PKC from macrophages may also change the membrane microviscosity and thus affect interaction with the parasites.

The present study was undertaken to investigate the relationship between generation of superoxide and activation and desensitisation of PKC in cultured macrophages. The role of membrane microviscosity of PKC-desensitised macrophages in the initial uptake of the parasites and the key role of superoxide in the multipliaton of the parasites were also studied.

6.2 Materials and Methods

6.2.1 Reagents

RPMI 1640 with L-glutamine, M199, and FCS were from GIBCO Laboratories, USA. Phorbol-12-myristate-13-acetate (PMA), staurosporine, phosphatidyl serine (PS), β–mercaptoethanol (ME), ethylene glycol tetraacetic acid (EGTA), phenyl methyl sulphonyl fluoride (PMSF), and histone IIIwere purchased from Sigma Chemical (St. Louis, MO). Tyrphostin AG126 was a generous gift from Prof. A Levitzki (Dept. of Biological Chemistry, the Hebrew Univ. of Jerusalem). Diphenyl hexatriene (DPH) and all other reagents used were of analytical grade.

6.2.2 Peritoneal Macrophages

Thioglycollate (TG)-elicited macrophages were isolated by peritoneal lavage from female Swiss albino mice. Four days after thioglycollate injection, macrophages were isolated by the method of Russel et al (283) from the peritoneal cavity, by washing with 3-4 ml of RPMI 1640 medium supplemented with 25 mM HEPES, 100 μg/ml streptomycin, 100 μg/ml penicillin and 20% of FCS. The macrophages were plated onto 18-mm coverslips and allowed to adhere at 37°C for 2 hr. Nonadherent cells were separated from macrophages by extensive washing of the coverslips with PBS. Cells obtained this way were ~85% viable as judged by trypan blue exclusion test.

6.2.3 Parasites

L.donovani AG83 (MHOM/IN/1983/AG83) and GE-1 (MHOM/lN/89/GE- 1) strains were maintained in female BALB/c mice. Parasites were recovered from the spleen of infected mice by adding spleens to culture medium M199 supplemented with 20% FCS, 100 μg/ml penicillin, and 100 μg/ml streptomycin. They were kept for 5 days at 22°C to obtain promastigotes, which were then washed and used for infection of macrophages.

6.2.4 Infection of Macrophages

Peritoneal macrophages were incubated with promastigotes for 2 hr at 37°C at a 10:1 parasite-to-cell ratio. Non-ingested parasites were removed by three washes with warm

PBS. Infection levels were determined by microscopic examination of Giemsa-stained coverslips.

6.2.5 Activation and Depletion of PKC in Macrophages

Macrophages were treated with 100 ng/ml or 1 µg/ml of PMA at 37°C for 45 min for activation of PKC (371). For depletion of PKC, cells were treated with 100 ng/ml PMA for 24 hr, washed three times, and resuspended in complete medium. This treatment specially depletes PKC activity in different systems (372).

6.2.6 Preparation of Membrane Fractions for PKC Assay

Cells from the TG-elicited mice macrophages were obtained after incubation for 2 hr at 37°C, then washed with PBS. After removing the nonadherent cells, the macrophages were stimulated for different times with PMA (100 ng/ml), then sonicated in buffer containing 0.25 mM sucrose, 5 mM EGTA, HEPES 20 mM, Leu-pep 50 µg/ml, PMSF 0.2 mM, and 2 mM β-mercaptoethanol. Thesonicate was centrifuged at 100,000 x g for 30 min. The pellet was resuspended in buffer supplemented with 1% (v/v) Triton-X 100 and centrifuged at 100,000 x g for 30 min. The detergent-treated supernatant fraction, i.e., the membrane fraction was assayed for PKC activity as described (373) using histoneIII as protein substrate. Briefly, PKC activity was measured as the incorporation of ^{32}P from ^{32}P ATP into histone Ill at 37°C in the presence of 10 mM $MgCl_2$, 50 µM ATP (containing approx. 6 X 10^5 cpm ^{32}P), 40 µg histone, 0.4 mM EGTA, 0.2 mM PMSF, 10mM 2ME, 0.01% Triton X-100, 1 mM $CaCl_2$, 20 µg/ml PS, and 2 µg/ml Diolein. Samples were assayed in duplicate in both the presence and absence of added Ca^{2+}, PS and diolein PKC activity was determined by subtracting from the maximal apparent activity the amount of ^{32}P incorporated into histone in the absence of essential cofactors and expressed as percentage (%) ^{32}P incorporation /mg of protein.

6.2.7 Membrane of PKC-Depleted Macrophages and Determination of Micro viscosity by Fluorescence Depolarization

Membranes of normal and PKC-depleted macrophages were isolated from other organelles by different centrifugation according to Werb et al. (374) and purified by discontinuous sucrose density gradient centrifugation. Fluidity of the macrophage membranes was determined by fluorescence depolarisation measurement using DPH as the probe (86). In short, DPH solution (2 mM) in THF was injected with rapid stirring into 1,000 volumes of PBS at room temperature. It was stirred for 2hr, then examined for negligible fluorescence. In experiments, both normal and PKC-depleted, macrophage membranes equivalent to 100 µg of cell protein were incubated in 2 ml of PBS containing 1 µM DPH preparation for 2-4 hr at 37°C with occasional stirring. Fluorescence intensity was measured in a fluorescence polarization spectrometer (PerkinElmer, SL-8) at room temperature with an excitation wavelength of 365 nm and an emission wavelength of 430 nm, and florescence anisotropy was calculated using the equation

$$r = (I_{\parallel} - I_{\perp}) / (I_{\parallel} + 2I_{\perp})$$

where $I_{\parallel}$ and $I_{\perp}$ are the fluorescence intensities oriented, respectively, parallel and perpendicular to the direction of polarization of the exciting light. The microviscosity parameters $[(r_0/r)-1]^{-1}$ were calculated in each case, knowing the fluorescence anisotropy r and the maximal limiting fluorescence anisotropy r_0, which for DPH was observed to have an experimental value of 0.362 (89). All measurements were performed within 24 hr after incubation.

6.2.8 Measurement of Superoxide of Activated and PKC-Depleted Macrophages

Superoxide anion generation by macrophages was determined at 37°C as previously described (375). Briefly, adherent cells on coverslips were washed thoroughly with PBS and placed in 35-mm diameter petridishes containing 1 ml of the reaction mixture. The reaction mixture contained 80 μM ferricytochrome c and 100 ng/ml PMA in phosphate buffer (pH 7.4) consisting of 137 mM NaCI, 2.7 mM KCl, 1.47 mM KH_2PO_4, 8.06 mM Na_2HPO_4, 0.8 mM $CaCI_2$, 0.4 mM $MgCI_2$, and 5.5 mM glucose, with or without 50 μg/ml superoxide dismutase (SOD). After incubation for 60 min at 37°C, O_2^- release was determined as SOD-inhibitable reduction of ferricytochrome c at 550 nm.

6.3 Results

6.3.1 Analysis of PMA-Pretreated Macrophage Uptake or Killing of Promastigotes of *L. donovani* AG83 and GE-1 Strains

To evaluate the role of PMA-pretreated macrophages in the process of infection by the parasites, we used TG-elicited peritoneal macrophages treated with PMA (100 ng/ml) for 45 min, 4 hr, or 24 hr. We examined the uptake by incubating the promastigote form of the parasites (strain AG83 or GE-I) with macrophage monolayers pre-treated with PMA for 4 or 24 hr at 37°C. Parasite uptake was assayed by light microscopy using Giemsa-stained slides (Table 6A₁). Uptake was found to be significantly higher for both the strains with macrophages pre-treated for 4 or 24 hr; approximately 30-40% more parasite uptake was found in 24 hr PMA-pretreated macrophages than in the nontreated macrophage control. In contrast, when macrophages were preincubated for 45 min with PMA, leishmanicidal activity of macrophages was observed, and approximately 40-50% parasites were killed by PMA-activated marophages (Table-6A₂). It is known that phorbol esters stimulate macropinocytosis and solute flow through macrophages (376) and here we show that they have diverse effects on *Leishmania* infection.

TABLE-6A: Effect of PMA-pretreatment of mouse peritoneal macrophages on the (6A1) uptake and (6A2) killing of *L. donovani* AG-83 and GE-1 promastigotes

(6A1) UPTAKE

Pretreatment[1]	Leishmania / 100 macrophages, 2 h after infection[2]		% Uptake	
	AG-83	GE-1	AG-83	GE-1
None	196 ± 6.0	301 ± 12.0		
PMA(4h)	321 ± 7.0	328 ± 7.0	119	109
PMA(24h)	277 ± 2.0	364 ± 6.0	142	121

(6A2) KILLING

Pretreatment[1]	Leishmania / 100 macrophages, 2 h after infection[2]		% Killing	
	AG-83	GE-1	AG-83	GE-1
None	194 ± 6.0	301 ± 12.0		
PMA(45 min)	121 ± 6.0	171 ± 7.0	48	43

[1]Untreated or PMA-pretreated (for indicated times) mouse peritoneal macrophages were incubated for 2h with AG-83 or GE-1 parasites in complete medium, washed, cultured for another 2h, washed, fixed, and stained as described in 'Materials and Methods'.
[2]These values represent the means ± S.D of these separate experiments performed with duplicate samples.

6.3.2 Activation and Depletion of PKC and Intracellular Fate of *Leishmania*

It has been shown that PMA, an agonist of PKC, activates or depletes PKC in different cell systems (371, 372) depending upon the time of treatment. The results of time-dependent PKC assay on normal and infected macrophage membranes are shown in Table 6B. Pretreatment with PMA for the shorter time (45 min) clearly promoted the activation of PKC, whereas longer (24 hr) preincubation with PMA led to its depletion. To test whether *Leishmania* killing or uptake by PMA-pretreated macrophages is PKC mediated, two approaches were taken. (i) Macrophages were incubated with inhibitors of PKC or tyrosine kinase. Inhibitors of kinases were used because it was thought that the killing of the parasite might be due to protein kinase-mediated O_2^- generation, and also because it is known that, in addition to the PKC-dependent phosphorylation of serine and threonine residues in specific proteins, the respiratory burst is accompanied by the phosphorylation of some proteins at tyrosine residues (234). Pretreatment of macrophages with staurosporine (0.1 μM, 10 min, 37°C), an inhibitor of PKC (390, 391), protected the parasites significantly, whereas tyrophostin AG126, a well-known inhibitor of protein tyrosine kinase (377) in macrophages, showed very little effect. Staurosporine protected the GE-I parasite significantly (approximately 85% of control parasites survived in staurosporine-treated macrophages) in PMA-activates (45 min treated) macrophages compared to control PMA-activated macrophages (Table 6C). (ii) PKC was depleted from macrophages by treatment with 100 ng/ml of PMA for 24 hr

(372) as described before. The depleted macrophages were then challenged with either AG83 or GE-I parasites. Table 6A indicates that 42±2.5 and 20±6.5% more uptake was found for AG-83 and GE-1 strains. Collectively, these results indicated that PMA pretreatment of macrophages contributed significantly towards the leishmanicidal activity or uptake of the parasites via a PKC-dependent mechanism.

TABLE-6B: Effects of PMA on specific activity of PKC in macrophage membrane protein

| Treatment | Histone phosphorylation (% 32P incorporation / mg of protein) in macrophage membrane fractions | | |
	Activated (% 32P inorporation/ mg of protein	Nonactivated (% 32P incorporation / mg protein	Actual 32P incorporation
Control	1.53	1.15	0.38
PMA (45 mm)	1.88	1.31	0.57
PMA(45min)+ L.*donovani* (AG-83)	1.61	1.14	0.47
PMA(24h)	0.92	0.75	0.17
PMA (24h) + *L.donovani* (AG-83)	0.78	0.69	0.09.

[1]Macrophages were incubated with or without *L. donovani* (AG-83) (for 2h in a cell: parasite ratio of 1:10), with or without pretreatment with PMA (100 ng/ml). PKC activities were assayed in membrane fractions.

TABLE-6C: Inhibitory effect of staurosporine or tyrphostin AG-126 on PMA-induced killing of *L.donovani* GE-1 parasites

Treatment[1]	*Leishmania*/ 100 macrophages[2] 2h after infection
None	303 ± 15.2
PMA	171± 7.0
Staurosporine + PMA	260 ± 8.02
Tyrphostin AG 126 + PMA	194 ± 6.55

[1]Staurosporine (0.1 µM for 10 min) or Tyrphostin AG-126 (20 µM for 2h) was added prior to the addition of PMA (100 ng/ml for 45 min). Macrophages were then infected for 2h and killing of the parasites was assessed by light microscopy.
[2]All values are mean ±S.D of duplicate samples.

6.3.3 Depletion of PKC Affects the Membrane Fluidity/Microviscosity of Macrophages

To examine whether membrane fluidity or microviscosity interferes with the parasite uptake by PKC-depleted macrophages, we isolated membranes from both normal and PKC-depleted macrophages. Membranes were incubated with the DPH probe at 37°C for 2 hr, then fluorescence was measured and microviscosity calculated (378). As shown in Table 6D, microviscosity of PKC-depleted macrophage membranes was found to be 0.7±0.05 (n=3), whereas that of normal was 1.16±0.10, indicating that the membrane of PKC-depleted macrophages was approximately 40% more fluid and thus possibly more permeable. The effects of variation in macrophage membrane microviscosity on the attachment and internalisation of *L. donovani* promastigotes was previously reported from this laboratory (378). In that report, we demonstrated that macrophage membrane fluidity or microviscosity significantly influences the attachment and internationalisation of parasites, and this influence may be causally related to the expression of receptors on the macrophage's surface. The increase in microviscosity (or decrease in fluidity) helps in receptor expression and, thus, the attachment of parasites.

TABLE-6D: Determination of membrane microviscosity of macrophages1 after prolonged treatment with PMA (PKC-depleted)

Membrane	Microviscosity parameters [(ro/r) - 1]-I 2
(i) Normal macrophages	1.16 ± 0.098
(ii) PKC-depleted macrophages	0.7 ± 0.045

[1]All values are means ± S.D (n=3).
[2]The microviscosity parameter was calculated from fluorescence depolarisation measurement using 1,3,5–diphenyl hexatriene as fluorescent probe.

On the contrary, an increase in fluidity (or decrease in microviscosity) does not increase parasite attachment, because of poor receptor expression, but expedites the process of compartmentalisation or invagination, which is a prerequisite for internalisation of parasites or endocytosis. In close agreement with the previous report, we show here that PKC-depleted macrophages internalise more parasites due to increased fluidity of their membranes. Previous studies with artificial and natural membranes have demonstrated the importance of lipid protein association in modulating the distribution of membrane proteins, membrane-fusion and membrane permeability (379).

6.3.4 Effect of PKC-Depletion on Intracellular Multiplication of *L.donovani* strains

Murray (380) showed that peritoneal macrophages pretreated for 2 hr with PMA had reduced leishmanicidal activity, indicating a role for PKC in the regulation of Leishmanial infection. Here we compared the uptake and multiplication of AG83 and GE-1 strains of *L. donovani* in PMA-pretreated peritoneal macrophages. Uptake of AG83 and GE-1 parasites/100 macrophages amounted to 231±7.0 and 328±7.0 in 4 hr PMA-pretreated cells, compared to 194±6.0 and 301±12.0 in non-treated cells whereas in 24 hr PMA-pretreated cells, the figures were 277±2.0 and 364±6.0 respectively. Thus, approximately 20% and 40% more uptake of GE-1 and AG83 parasites was found in 24 hr PMA-treated macrophages. The effect of 24 hr PMA pretreatment was also determined on the multiplication of parasites. As shown in Figure 6A, 24 hr after infection, PMA-pretreated macrophages contained 40% more AG83 and 29% more GE-I (Fig.6B) than control, and by 48 hr, PMA-pretreated macrophages contained 52% more AG83 and 53% more GE-I than control.

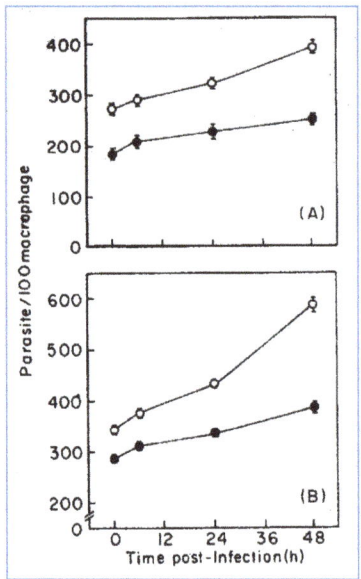

FIG. 6:   Intracellular multiplication of AG-83 or GE-I parasites in PKC-depleted macrophages. Untreated (closed symbols) and PMA-pretreated (open symbols) macrophages were infected with parasites as described in "Materials and Methods" and parasites survival was assessed at the indicated times. A, AG-83 promastigotes; B, GE-I promastigies. Each point represents the mean ± S.D of triplicate samples.

6.3.5 Superoxide of Activated and PKC-depleted Macrophages

Because PMA activates both the respiratory burst and PKC, superoxide generation was measured both in PMA-induced and PKC-depleted macrophages. TG-elicited peritoneal macrophages were tested for superoxide anion production after incubation for 1 hr with PMA in Kreb's Ringer phosphate glucose (KRPG). O_2^- production was increased by at least 3-fold compared with controls when macrophages were pretreated for 45 min with PMA (Table-6E). In contrast, the production of O_2^- was significantly reduced to far below the basal level in PKC-depleted macrophages. These results indicated that O_2^- might interfere with the killing and multiplication of parasites inside macrophages.

TABLE-6E: Production of superoxide anion by control and PMA-activated or PKC-depleted macrophages

Cell treatment[1]	O_2^- nmol/h/mg of protein[2]
None	87± 7.5
PMA (45min)	276 ± 25.2
PMA (24h)	47 ± 6.8

[1]Macrophage monolayers were prepared on coverslips as described in 'Materials and Methods'. Triplicate sets of macrophages were untreated or incubated with PMA for 45 min or 24hr, washed, then incubated with PMA containing KRPG for assay of O_2^-.
[2]Mean ± S.D of triplicate determinations for each treatment group.

6.4 Discussion

Infection of monocytes or macrophages with *Leishmania* attenuates PMA-stimulated oxygen consumption (323) and inhibits PKC-mediated events such as chemotactic locomotion (312) and c-fos gene expression (188). Although these observations indicate the involvement of PKC-mediated events in intact cells, there was no previous report on the activation and deactivation of PKC in macrophages and their role in degradation or survival of the parasites during infection. Therefore, in this study, we have investigated the effect of activation or depletion of PKC on uptake, multiplication, and degradation of two virulent strains of *L. donovani*.

It has been reported that depending upon the time of pre-treatment with PMA, macrophages activate or deplete PKC in intact cells (371, 380). It is known that PMA pretreatment for a longer period causes long lasting depletion of PKC isoforms in many biological systems (380). In our experiment, when the cells were pretreated with PMA for 45 min, 40-45% parasites were killed; but when the cells were preincubated with staurosporine, a potent inhibitor of PKC, parasites were protected (Table 6C). On the other hand, Tyrphostin AG126, an inhibitor of tyrosine kinase had little effect on the protection. Pretreatment of macrophages with PMA for 24 hr depletes PKC activity by increasing its rate of degradation (381). We found that the initial uptake of both AG83 and GE-I was significantly higher in PMA-pretreated macrophages than in non-treated cells. This suggests that phorbol ester-sensitive PKC depletion helps in the ingestion of *L.donovani* promastigotes, and this result is in agreement with the previous report by Murray (380). During the first 48 hr of infection, we found that PKC-depleted macrophages contained more parasites than normal macrophages. This enhanced growth in PMA-pretreated macrophages was evidenced further when we compared the multiplication of the parasites in normal and treated macrophages (Fig.6A, B). Collectively, these findings provide evidence that PKC-dependent events played a significant role in the proliferation of *L. donovani* inside macrophages. Although LPG from *L.donovani* promastigotes (382), and glycosylinositolphospholipids (342) from amastigotes were shown to be potent inhibitors of purified PKC *in vitro*, there might be a possibility that these types of molecules might down-regulate or deplete PKC activity in intact macrophages. The initial uptake of the parasites in PKC-depleted macrophages was higher than in normal macrophages, indicating the possibility of alteration of membrane fluidity or the microviscosity of macrophages. Our present data on membrane microviscosity showed that PKC-depleted macrophages are approximately 1.6-fold more fluid than the normal macrophages. This finding clearly indicates that whatever the exact mechanism of uptake might be, the fluidity or microviscosity of the membrane has a significant effect on the process, and this decrease in microviscosity or increase in fluidity may up- or down-regulate the expression of *Leishmania* recognition receptors. This result is in close agreement with the previous finding by Mukherjee et al. (378) that the microviscosity of the macrophage membrane is inversely collected with the number of parasites that are internalized. Though the exact molecular mechanism of higher uptake of the parasites is not clearly understood, it has been shown that modulation of artificial and natural membranes seems to affect the activity of many membrane-bound enzymes, the distribution of membrane proteins, membrane permeability and membrane fusion (379).

PMA activates both the respiratory burst and PKC in phagocytic cells (383, 384). The mechanism by which intracellular *Leishmania* interferes with the oxidative mechanism of host cells is unknown. To examine the relationship between PKC, O_2 generation, and the intracellular fate of *Leishmania* parasites, we tested the O_2 generation in PMA-induced (activated) and PKC-depleted macrophages. It is noteworthy that PMA (45 min) induced a significant amount of O_2 generation in macrophages and killed both AG83 and GE-I at the level of 40 and 45% respectively (Tables 6C, D); but killing was inhibited when macrophages were preincubated with staurosporine, an inhibitor of PKC. Indeed, staurosporine inhibited the PMA-induced oxidative burst and helped in the survival of the parasites. On the other hand, depletion of PKC drastically reduced the O_2 generation and facilitated the intracellular multiplication of the parasites. These data collectively suggest that PKC and O_2 are the major factors in parasite degradation and multiplication inside macrophages, although a recent report found altered activation and translocation of PKC in *Leishmania* infected human monocytes (237).

PKC is a key enzyme involved in the regulation and functions of many cell types via phosphorylation of its substrate proteins. For example, activation of neutrophils by several agents, including phorbol esters, results in phosphorylation of PKC-dependent proteins that are involved in superoxide anion production. A similar mechanism might be operative in the present study of PKC activation and O_2 generation in macrophàges, as shown by parasite killing and multiplication. It has been shown in bone marrow-derived macrophages that LPG of *L. donovani* inhibited the phosphorylation of MARCKS (myristoylated alanire-rich C kinase substrate), a well-known substrate of PKC (313), but whether this inhibition is related with O_2^- generation and multiplication of the parasites remains to be determined. In this connection, it is interesting to note that in CGD (chronic granulomatous disease) neutrophils fail to express a respiratory burst due to failure in PMA-induced phosphorylation of a 48kDa cytosolic protein (338).

In conclusion, our findings suggest that activation and depletion or inhibition of PKC of host macrophages regulates Leishmanial infection, atleast for the two virulent strains we examined. Although it is known that the depletion of PKC may alter various host functions, in the present report we show that down-regulation of membrane microviscosity and superoxide generation of PKC-depleted macrophages might facilitate the uptake and multiplication of the parasites.

SUMMARY

Antileishmanial therapy is still a very complicated subject because of the complexities of the disease and the inadequacy of published information. In addition to the conventional therapy as an alternative approach, people are now trying to exploit several surface receptors of host cells, eg., macrophages for activation purposes to fight against this deadly parasite, *L.donovani*, the etiological agent of visceral Leishmaniasis. We, therefore, thought that attempt could be made to control *Leishmania* infection either by modulating the surface receptor of macrophage or by identifying the signaling molecules generated e.g. kinases during early phases of *L. donovani*-macrophage interaction (Ligand-receptor interaction). Identifying these types of molecules would lead to design suitable inhibitors for blocking the infection.

Mannosyl-fucosyl receptor is a well-characterized receptor on the macrophage surface and this receptor has some definite role in the interaction process. We thus examined the attachment and internalisation of virulent and avirulent *L.donovani* promastigotes by macrophage MFR in the presence of oxidants and anti-inflammatory steroid dexamethasone. Oxidant and dexamethasone are known to down- and up-regulate the expression of MFR. Macrophages, when treated with 500 µM H_2O_2 at 37°C for 30 min, stimulate about 45% inhibition in the uptake of an avirulent strain UR6, and 30% and 25% inhibition of virulent strains AG-83 and GE-I, respectively. Treatment of macrophages with dexamethasone for 20h resulted in stimulation in the uptake of the parasite. When UR6 was used, a 3-fold increase in the uptake was observed compared to the controls. Parasite uptake was also inhibited by the H_2O_2-genarating system, glucose/ glucose oxidase, inhibition was blocked by catalase. Treatment of macrophages either with H_2O_2 or dexamethasone did not affect the binding of the advanced glycosylation end product bovine serum albumin (AGE-BSA), the ligand for AGE receptor of macrophages. Similarly, indirect evidence also shows that both types 1 and 3 complement receptors (CR1, CR3) are not affected by these treatments. Thus, the results suggest that *in vitro* modulation of the mannose-receptor affected the attachment and internalisation of both virulent and avirulent *L.donovani* promastigotes significantly **(Chapter 2)**.

L. donovani also interacts with macrophages via integrin receptors, which are involved in various kinds of cell signalling. To identify the signalling molecules responsible in the interaction process, we showed that protein tyrosine kinases also protein tyrosine phosphatases are involved in the uptake of virulent and avirulent *L. donovani* promastigotes by macrophage cells. Uptake inhibition assays with protein tyrosine kinase inhibitors, genistein or tyrphostin 25 decreased parasites' invasion in a dose-dependent manner, however, addition of sodium orthovanadate, a protein tyrosine phosphatase inhibitor, prior to infection, significantly increased parasite internalisation. A similar uptake profile was observed with both virulent and avirulent *L. donovani* promastigotes. Treatment of macrophages with cytochalasin B, an inhibitor of actin polymerisation, prevented the promastigote uptake - indicating probably tyrosine kinase induced actin polymerisation signal is necessary for the entry of the parasites, like the bacterial entry into mammalian systems. In contrast, neither genistein nor tyrphostin significantly reduced intracellular replication of this pathogen and nitric oxide production, suggesting PTK-mediated signal is not related to ultimate virulence mechanism associated with intracellular replication of this pathogen. We propose that invasion of both virulent and avirulent *L.donovani* promastigotes initiate a host cell PTK-dependent response signals for actin polymerisation and thus facilitates the phagocytosis **(Chapter-3).**

In continuation of identifying various cell signalling molecules, we have investigated next, the role of Protein Kinase C (PKC) in oxidative events of macrophages infected with three different strains, GE-I, AG-83 and UR6 of *L.donovani* promastigotes. The oxidative events were compared with the macrophages that were allowed to attach with the parasite surface in the presence of a drug, cytochalasin D. *In vitro* replication studies inside macrophages and our, previous *in vivo* infection study showed that degree of virulency of the strains were in the following order: GE-I > AG-83 > UR6. Phorbol 12-myristate 13-acetate (PMA)-induced oxidative burst activity, and bacterial lipopolysaccharide plus interteron-γ (LPS + IFN-γ) induced NO production were markedly attenuated in macrophages infected with GE-I and AG-83 strains as compared to UR6. However, under parasite attachment condition, for all three strains, augmentation of O_2 Consumption, O_2^- generation and NO production was observed. Induction of O_2^- generation was inhibited by staurosporine, an inhibitor of PKC and NO production by staurosporine and PTK inhibitors, genistein and tyrphostin, indicating the role of PKC and PTK in parasite-mediated NO-signalling pathway. Together, these results suggest that although attachment of *L. donovani* parasites like any other microorganism induced PKC-mediated oxidative events, these events are significantly down-regulated in macrophages after infection with GE-I or AG-83 strains, which may help in the parasite survival and multiplication and thus may contribute to chronic infection **(Chapter-4).**

Next, we demonstrated incorporation of exogeneously added [^{32}P] orthophosphate or [^{3}H] myristic acid into specific macrophage proteins during attachment of the cells with virulent strains (AG-83, GE-I) of *L. donovani* promastigotes. Cytochalasin D, an inhibitor of actin polymerisation was used to inhibit uptake of parasites by macrophages. Attachment of the promastigotes to the cells induced the phosphorylation of the proteins with molecular mass of 29- and 45 kDa. Addition of phorbol 12 myristate 13 acetate (PMA) further induced the phosphorylations. Staurosporine, an inhibitor of PKC blocked the phosphorylations of these proteins. However, phosphorylations of these proteins were significantly down-regulated when macrophages were infected with the virulent strains of the promastigotes for approximately 48-72 hrs. Phosphorylations of these proteins did not occur when the cells were allowed to attach with other intramacrophage pathogens such as *E. coli* or *Shigella flexneri* indicating that *L.donovani* specific signals are induced in phosphorylation. Interestingly, attachment of *L.donovani* promastigotes also induced the myristoylation of a 29 kDa protein and a protein in the region of 42-45 kDa, and myristoylations of these proteins were further induced when the cells were preincubated with bacterial LPS or conA-stimulated T-cell supernatant indicating that *L.donovani* attachment could not suppress LPS or IFN-γ mediated signalling. Together, these data suggest that induced PKC-mediated phosphorylations and myristoylation signals are *L. donovani* attachment specific and this signal differs significantly with intracellular replication of the parasites **(Chapter-5).**

Finally, we also showed that PKC is not only involved in attachment and entry process but also regulates intracellular replication of this parasite. Thus, pre-treatment of macrophages with PMA, an agonist of PKC, showed diverse effects on degradation and survival of two virulent strains of *Leishmania donovani* promastigotes. Treatment of macrophages with PMA for 45 min at 37°C generated significant amount of superoxide anions and reduced the parasite burden of macrophages by 48% and 43% respectively when AG83 and GE-I strains were used for infection. Staurosporine, an inhibitor of PKC, inhibited PMA-dependent killing of the parasites, while tyrphostin AG-126, an inhibitor of protein tyrosine kinase, showed very little effect. Depletion of PKC by prolonged incubation with PMA drastically reduced the superoxide anion generation and increased the uptake and multiplication of the parasites. Finally, to understand the mechanism of higher uptake of the parasites by PKC-depleted macrophages, membrane microviscosity was measured by fluorescence depolarization. Membrane microviscosity was found to be approximately 40% lower in PKC-depleted macrophages than that in the normal macrophages, indicating the role of membrane fluidity in the infection process. Together, these data suggest that PKC activation, superoxide generation, and membrane fluidity are essential factors in the efficient regulation of Leishmanial infection. As we observed that depletion of PKC induced the intracellular multiplication of the parasites at least for two virulent strains GE-I and AG83 **(Chapter-6),** designing and synthesis of suitable PKC inhibitors could help us to block the entry process.

Thus, signal transduction based measures provide alternative approaches to control visceral leishmaniasis.

REFERENCES

1. Sanyal RK (1985). Leishmaniasis in human parasitic diseases (Chang KP and Bray RS eds.) Elsevier Publishers, p442-

2. Chang KP, Fong D and Bray RS (1985), Leishmaniasis in human parasitic diseases (Chang KP and Bray RS eds.), Elsevier Publishers, p2-

3. Locksley RM, Heinzel FP, Fankhauser JE, Nelson CS, Sadick MD (1988). Infect Immun. **56**: p336-

4. Zuckerman A and Lainson R (1977). Parasitic Protozoa (Kreier JP ed.). Academic Press, New York, Sanfrancisco, London, p57-

5. Bray RS (1974). Annu. Rev. Microbio, **28**: p189-

6. Dwyer DM and Gottlieb M (1983). J. Cell Biochem. **23**: p35-

7. Adler S (1964), Adv. Parasitol. **2**: p35-

8. Herrer A (1971), J. Parasitol. **57**: p626-

9. Kellina 01(1962). Med. Parasitol Bolezni. **31**: p716-

10. Roberts LS, Janovy J Jr. (2000). Foundations of Paraitology, 6th International Ed.

11. Kane MM, Mosser DM (2000). Curr. Opin. Hematol. **7:** p26-

12. Chatterjee KD (1975). Human parasites and parasitic diseases, Saraswati Press, Calcutta, India

13. Chang KP and Fish WR (1983). In vitro cultivation of Protozoan parasites (Jenson JB ed.), CRC Press, Florida, p112-

14. Battaglia PA, Bue Mdel, Ottaviano M, Ponzi M (1983). Molecular biology of parasites, New York: Raven Press, p107.

15. Stuart K (1983). Mol. Biochem. Parasitol. **9:** p93-

16. Rabinovitch M, Topper G, Cristello P, Rich A (1985). J. Leukoc. Biol. **37:**p247-

17. Peters C, Aebischer T, Stierhof YD, Fuchs M, Overath P (1995) J. Cell Sci.**108**: p3715-

18. Dwyer DM, Gottlieb M (1985). Leishmaniasis in human parasitic diseases. (Chang KP and Bray RS eds.), Elsevier Science Publishers, p32-

19. Dwyer DM (1974) Science **184:** p471-

20. Hernandez AG, Arguello C, Ayesta C, Dagger F, Infante RB, Stojanovich D, Dawidowicz K, Riggione F, La Riva G (1981). Biochemistry of Parasites (Slutzky GM ed.), Pergamon Press, Oxford, p48-

21. Dwyer DM (1977). Exp. Parasitol **41**: p341

22. Jacobson RL, Slutzky GM, Greenblatt CL, Schnur LF (1982). Annu, Trop. Med. Parasitol **76**: p45-

23. Dawidowicz K, Hernandez AG, Infante RB (1975). J. Parasitol, **61**: p950-

24. Descoteaux A, Turco SJ (1999). Biochim. Biophys. Acta. **1455:** p341-

25. Marr JJ (1984). Parasitic Diseases (Mansfield JM ed.), Marcel Dekker Inc. New York and Basel, p201-

26. Goad IJ, Holz GG, Beach DH (1984). Mol. Biochem. Parasitol. **10:** p161-

27. Hernandez AG, Rascon A, Kutner S, Roman H and Campos Z (1993). Mol. Biol. Reports, **18:** p189-

28. Doyle PS and Dwyer DM (1993). Exp. Parasitol **77:** p435-

29. Gottlieb M (1989). Parasitol. Today **5:** p257-

30. Kelleher M, Bacic A, Handman E (1992). Proc. Natl. Acad. Sci. USA., **89:** p6-

31. Bahr V, Stierhof YD, Ilg T, Demar M, Quinten M, Overath P (1993). Mol. Biochem. Parasitol. **53:** p107-

32. Mareden P (1979). N. Eng. J. Med. **300:** p350

33. Pearson RD (1993). Immunology and molecular biology of parasitic infections. Boston: Blackwell scientific Pub (Warren KS ed.)

34. World Health Organization Expert Committee, WHO Technical Report Series 701, (1984). WHO, Geneva.

35. Locksley RM, Louis JA (192). Curr. Opin. in Immunol. **4:** p413-

36. Mauel J and Behin R (1982). Immunology of parasitic infections. Oxford: Blackwell Scientific Publication Ltd. p299-

37. Modabber F (1990). TDR news, UNDP/World Bank/WHO special programme for research and training in tropical diseases No. **34:** p1-

38. Auger MJ and Ross JA (1992). The Macrophage (Lewis CE and McGee JO'D. ed.), IRL Press, Oxford, New york, Tokyo, p1-

39. Coleman RM, Lombard MF and Sicard RE (1989). Fundamental Immunology (Wheatley CH et.), Wm. C. Brown Publishers, USA, p205-

40. Werb Z (1982). Basic and Clinical Immunology (Stites DP, Stobo JD, Fudenberg HH and Wells JV eds.), Large Medical Publications, Los Atlos, California, p110-

41. van Furth R and Sluitar W (1986). J. Exp. Med. **163:** p474-

42. Simon LM, Robin ED, Phillips JR, Acevedo J, Axline SG and Theodore J (1977), J. Clin. Invest. **59:**p443.

43. Pierce CW and Kapp JA (1976). Immunobiology of the Macrophage (Nelson DS ed.), Academic Press, New York, Sanfrancisco, London, p7-

44. Vaux D and Gordon S (1981). Methods for studying Mononuclear Phagocytes (Adams DO and Koren HS ed.), Academic Press, New York.

45. Zuckerman SH and Douglas SD (1979). Annu. Rev. Microbiol. **33:** p269-

46. Lockwood BC, North MJ, Mallinson DJ and Coombs GH (1987). Ferns. Microbiol. Lett. **48:** p345-

47. Adams DO and Hamilton TA (1984). Annu. Rev. Immunol. **2:** p283-

48. Steinmann RM and Cohn ZA (1974). Inflammatory Process (Zweifach BW, Grant L and McCluskey RT ed.), Academic Press, New York, p449-

49. Cohn ZA (1978). J. Immunol. **121:** p813-

50. Nathan CF, Silverstein SC, Brukner LH and Cohn ZA (1979). J. Exp. Med. **149:** 100-

51. Ezekowitz RAB, Austyp J, Stahl PD and Gordon S (1981). J. Exp. Med. **154**:p60-

52. Johnston RB Jr., Godzik CA and Cohn ZA (1978). J. Exp Med. **148**: p115-

53. Edeison PJ (1981). Lymphokines. **3**: p57-

54. Nathan C and Cohn ZA (190). J. Exp. Med. **152:** p183-

55. Adams DO, Kao KJ, Farb R and Pizzo SV (1980). J. lmmunol. **124**: p298-

56. Marino P and Adams DO (1980). Cell Immunol. **54**: p11-

57. Imber MJ, Pizzo SV, Johnson WJ and Adams DO (1982). J. Biol. Chem. **257**: p5129-

58. Lane FC and Unanue ER (1972). J. Exp. Med. **135**: p1104-

59. North RJ (1973) J. Exp. Med. **138:** p342-

60. Dumonde C, Wolstencroft RA, Panayo GS, Mathew M, Morley J and Howson WT (1969). Nature (London) **224**: p38-

61. Buchmuller -Rouiler Y and Mauel J (1979). J. Exp. Med. **150**: p359-

62. Scott CL, Roe L, Curtis J, Baldwin T, Robb L, Begley CG, Handman E (2000). Microbes Infect **2:** p1131-

63. Roitt I, Brostoff J, Male D (1996). Immunology, 4th Ed. Times Mirror International Publishers Ltd.

64. David JR and Remold HG (1976). Immunobiology of the macrophage (Nelson DS ed.), Academic Press, New York, p401-

65. Karnovsky ML and Lazdins JK (1978) J. Immunol. **121**: p809-

66. Ogmundsdottir HM and weir DM (1980). Clin. Exp. Lmmunol. **40**: p223-

67. Walker WS (1977). J.Immunol. **119**: p367-

68. Capron A, Dessaint JP, Joseph M, Rousseaux R, Capron M and Bazin H (1977). Eur. J. Immunol. **7**: p315-

69. Pestel J, Joseph M, Dessaint JP and Capron A (1980). In 4th International Congress of Immunology. Abstract 7.1.13.

70. Alexander P and Evans R (1971). Nature **232**: p76-

71. Arauzo FG and Remington JS (1974). Immunology, **27**: p711-

72. Watnick AS and Gordon AS (1964). J. Reticuloendothel. Soc. **1**: p170-

73. Nelson DS (1972). Critical Reviews of Microbiology (I), CRS Press, Cleveland p353-

74. Schorlemmer HV and Allison AC (1976). Immunol. **31**: p781-

75. Ferluga I, Schorlemmer HV, Baptista LC and Allison AC (1978). Clin. Exp. Immunol. **31**: p512-

76. Davies JW, Lowrie DB and Cole PJ (1995). J. Immunol. **154:** p1909-

77. Edwards III CK, Ghiasuddin SM, Schepper JM, Yunger LM and Kelley KW (1988). Science **239:** p769-

78. Douglas SD and Hassan NF (1990). Haematology (Williams WJ, Beutler E, Erslev AJ and Lichtman MA ed.). McGraw-Hill, New York.

79. Carr L (1973). The macrophage. A review of ultrastructure and function, Academic Press, London, p10-

80. Kaplan G (1977). Scan J. Immurtol. **6:** p797-

81. Orenstein JM and Shelton E (1977). Lab. Invest, **36**: p363-

82. Reaven EP and Axline SG (1973). J. Cell Biol. **59**: p12-
83. Ezekowitz RAB and Gordon S (1982). J Exp Med. **155:** p1623-
84. Lewis DH and Peters W (1977). Annu. Trop.Med. Parasitol. **71:** p295-
85. Borochov H and Shinitzky M (1976). Proc. Natl. Acad. Sci. USA, **73:** p4526-
86. Basu MK, Flamm M, Schachter D, Bertles JF, Maniasis A (1980). Biochem. Biophys. Res. Comm. **95**: p887-
87. Shinitzky M and Souroujon M (1979). Proc. Nati. Acad. Sci,USA., **76**: p4438-
88. Hilderbrand JH (1972). Proc. Natl. Acad. Sci. USA. **69**: p3428-
89. Shinitzky M and Bernholz Y (1974). J. Biol. Chem. **249**: p2652-
90. Schachter D and Shinitzky M (1977). J. Clin. Invest. **59**: p536-
91. Unanue R (1981).Adv. Immunol. **31**: p1-
92. Bellier DI and Unanue ER (1982). Lymphokines (Mizel S ed.), Academic Press, New York, p25-
93. Springer T, Galfre G, Secher DS and Milstein C (1979). Eur. J. immunol. **9:** 301-
94. Borges MM, Campos Neto A, Sleath P, Grabstein KH, Morrissey PJ, Skeiky YA, Reed SG (2001). Infect. Immun. **69:** p5270-
95. Chakraborty R, Chakraborty P, Basu MK (1998). Bioscience Report, **18**: p129-
96. Chang KP (1981). Mol. Biochem. Parasitol. **4:** p67-
97. Blackwell JM (1985). Trans. R. Soc. Trop. Med. Hyg. **79:** p606-
98. Banerjee G, Nandi G, Mahato SB, Pakrashi A and Basu MK (1996). J. Antimicrobiol. Chemo **38**: p145-
99. Banerjee G, Medda S, Basu MK (1998). Antimicrobial. Agents and Chemo. **42**: p348-
100. Taylor ME (1993) Biochem. Soc. Trans. **21**: p468-
101. Haitiwanger RS, Hill RL (1986). J. Biol. Chem **261**: p15696-
102. Chakraborty P, Das PK (1988). Mol. Biochem. Parasitol. **28:** p55-
103. Kahn S, Wleklinski M, Ezekowitz RA, Coder D, Aruffo A, Farr A (1995). J. Exp. Med. **182**: p1243-
104. Taylor ME, Drickamerk (1993). Annu. Rev. Cell Biol. **9**: p237-
105. Channon JY, Roberts MB, Blackwell JM (1984). Immunology **53**: p345-
106. Stahl PD, Rodman JS, Miller MJ, Schlesinger PH (1978). Proc. Natl. Acad. Sci. USA., **75**: p1399-
107. Noorman F, Braat EA, Rijken DC (1995). Blood. **86**: p3421-
108. Mokaena T, Gordon S (1985). J. Clin. Invest. **75**: p624-
109. Bozeman PM, Hoidal JR, Shepherd VL (1988). J. Biol. Chem. **263**: p1240-
110. Taylor ME, Bezouska and Drickamar K (1992). J. Biol. Chem. **267**: p:1719-
111. Engering AJ, Cella M, Fluitsma DM and Hoefsmit EC, Lanzavecchia A, Pieters J (1997). Adv. Exp. Med. Biol. **417**: p183
112. Ohsumi Y and Lee YC (1987). J. Biol. Chem. **262**: p7955-
113. Klegeris A, Budd TC and Greenfield SA (1996). Biochim. Biophys. Acta. **1289**: p159-
114. Shibata Y, Metzger WJ, Myrvik QN (1997). J. Immunol. **159:** p2462-
115. Yamamoto Y, Klein TW and Friedman H (1997). Infect. Immun. **65:** p1077-

116. Hynes RO (1992). Cell **69**: p11-

117. Leong JM, Fournier RS and lsberg RR (1991) Infect. Immun. **59**: p3424-

118. Leong JM, Fournier RS and Isberg RR (1990). Infect. Immun. **59**: p3424-

119. Bliska JB, Galan JE and Falkow S (1993). Cell **73**: p903-

120. Wright SD, Reddy PA, Jong MT, Erikson BW (1987). Proc. NatI. Acad. Sci, USA. **84:** p1965-

121. Russel DG and Wright SD (1988). J. Exp. Med. **168:** p279-

122. Bray RS, Alexander J (1982). Leishmaniasis in Biology and Medicine, Academic Press, London.

123. Walker WS and Yen SE (1982). J. Cell Physiol. **110**: p277-

124. Rosenthal LA, Sutterwala FS, Kehrli ME, Mosser DM (1996). Infec Immun. **64**:p2206-

125. Mosser DM, Edelson PJ (1985). J Immunol, **135**: p2785-

126. Da Silva RP, Hall BF, Joiner KA and Sacks DL (1989). J. Immunol. **143**: p617-

127. Mosser DM and Edelson PJ (1987). Nature. **327**: p329-

128. Mosser DM, Burke SK, Coutavas EE, Wedgwood JF and Edelson PJ (1986). Exp. Parasitol. **62**: p394-

129. Puentes SM, Dwyer DM, Bates PA, Joiner KA (1989). J. Immunol. **143**: p3743-

130. Hibino Y, Mariano TM, Kumar CS, Kozak CA, Pestka S (1991). J. Biol. Chem, **266**: p6948-

131. Singer SJ and Nicolson GL (1972). Science **175**: p720-

132. Klempner MS, Cendron M, Wyler DJ (1983). J. Infect. Dis. **148:** p377-

133. Chang KP, Fong D (1983). Cytopathology of Parasitic Diseases, Pitman Books, London, p113-

134. Brown CC and Gallin JI (1988). Haematology/Oncology. clinics of North America, Phagocytic Defects, Vol.1 (Curnutte, JT ed.). WB Saunders, Philadelphia. **2**: p61-

135. Mauel J (1984). Parasitol **88**: p579-

136. Chang KP, Fong D and Chaudhuri G (1990). Annu. Rev. Microbiol. **44**: p499-

137. Thorne KJ and Blackwell JM (1983). Adv Parasitol **22**: p43-

138. Blackwell JM and Alexander J (1983). Trans. Soc. Trop. Med. Hyg. **77**:p636-

139. Metcalf D (1971) J. Cell. Physiol. **77**: p277-

140. Murray HW, Rubin BY and Rothermel CD (1983). J. Clin. Invest. **72**: p1506-

141. Murray HW (1990) J. Infect. Dis. **161**: p992-

142. Nathan CF, Murray HW, Wiebe ME and Rubin BY (1983). J Exp. Med. **158**: p670-

143. Scott P, Pearce E, Cheever AW, Coffman RL and Sher A (1989). lmmunol. Rev. **112**: p161-

144. Bogdan C, Moll H, Solbach W and Rollinghoff M (1990). Eur. J. Immunol **20**: p1131-

145. Green SJ, Meltzer MS, Hibbs JB (Jr) and Nacy CA (1990). J. Immunol, **144**:p278-

146. Green SJ, Crawford RM, Hockmeyer JT, Meltzer MS, Nacy CA (1990). J. Immunol. **145**: p4290-

147. Adams LB, Hibb JB (Jr), Tainter RR, Krahenbuhl JL (1990). J. Immunol.**144:** p2725-

148. Liew FY, Li Y and Millot S (1990). Immunol. **71**: p556-

149. Liew FY, Li Y and Millot S (1990). J. Immunol. **145:** p4306-

150. Sadick MD. Macrophage in parasite infection. In: The Natural Immune System. The Macrophage by Lewis EC and McGee OD. James Ed. IRL Press. Oxford Univ. p 265-

151. Liew FY, Millot S, Parkinson C, Palmer RM and Moncada S (1990). J. Immunol. **144:** p4794-

152. Murray HW(1981a). J. Exp. Med. **153:** p1302-

153. Roach TI, Kiderlen AF and Blackwell JM (1991). Infect. Immun. **59:** p3935-

154. Anon (1990). World Report on Tropical Disease. WHO.

155. Severn A, Xu D, Doyle J, Leal LM, O'Donnell CA, Brett SJ, Moss DW, Liew FY (1993). Eur, J. Immunol. **23:** p566-

156. Liew FY (1989). Immunol. Today. **10:** p40-

157. Scott P and Sher A (1986). J. Immunol. **136:** p1461-

158. Mauel J (1990). J. Leukoc. Biol. **47:** 187-

159. Hockertz S, Baccarin M and Lohman-Mathes ML (1989). J. Immunol. **142:** p2489-

160. Snyderman R and Pike MC (1984). Annu. Rev. Immunol. **2:** p257-

161. Fearson DT (1980). J. Exp. Med. **52:** p20-

162. Chang KP (1983). Int. Rev Cytol. Suppl. **14:** p267-

163. Mosser DM and Edelson PJ (1984). J. Immunol. **132:** p1501-

164. Blackwell JM, Ezekowitz RA, Roberts MB, Channon JY, Sim RB and Gordon S (1985). J. Exp. Med **162:** p324-

165. Wilson ME and Pearson RD (1988). Infect. Immun. **56:** p363-

166. Wright SD, Weitz JI, Huang AJ, Levin SM, Silverstein SL, Loike JD (1988). Proc. NatI. Acad. Sci., USA. **85:** p7734-

167. Wright SD and Jong MT (1986). J. Exp. Med. **164:** p1876-

168. Myones BL, Dalzell JG, Hogg N and Ross GD (1988). J. Clin. Invest. **82:** p640-

169. Dustin ML and Springer TA (1988). J. Cell Biol **107:** p321-

170. Murray HW (1981b). J. Exp. Med. **153:** p1690-

171. Gehlsen KR, Dillner L, Engvall E and Rouslahti E (1988). Science **241:** p1228-

172. Wayner EA and Carter WG (1987). J. Cell Biol, **105:** p1873-

173. Wilson ME, Hardin KK (1988), J. Immunol. **141:** p265-

174. Looney RJ, Abraham GN and Anderson CL (1986). J. Immunol. **136:** p1641-

175. Wileman TE, Lennartz MR and Stahl PD (1986). Proc. Natl. Acad. Sci., USA. **83:** p2501-

176. Vlassara H, Brownlee M and Cerami A (1984). J. Exp. Med. **160:** p197-

177. Wilson ME, Pearson RD (1986). J. lmmunol. **136:** p4681-

178. Chakraboy P, Ghosh D, Basu MK (2001). J. Parasitol. **87:** p1023-

179. Russell DG and Talamus-Rohana P (1989). Immunol. Today **10:** p328-

180. Turco SJ (1988). Biochem Soc Trans **16:** 259-

181. Handman E and Goding JW (1985). EMBO J. **4:** p329-

182. King DL, Chang YD and Turco SJ (1987). Mol. Biochem. Parasitol. **24:** p47-

183. Etges R, Bouvier J and Bordier C (1986). J Biol. Chem **261:** p9098-

184. Chang CS and Chang KP (1986) Proc. Natl. Acad. Sci. USA, **83:** p100-

185. Grimm F, Jenni L, Bouvier J, Etges RJ, Bordier C (1987). Acta. Trop. **44**: p375-

186. Dermine JF, Scianimanico S, Prive L, Descoteaux A, Desjardins M (2000). Cellular Microbiology. **2**: p115-

187. Wright EP, el Amin ER (1989). Biochem.Cell Biol. **67**: p525-

188. Descoteaux A, Turco SJ, Sacks DL, Matlashewski G (1991). J. Immunol. **146**: p2747-

189. Brittingham A, Morrison CJ, McMaster WR, McGwire 8S, Chang KP, Mosser DM (1995). J. Immunol. **155**: p3102-

190. Silverstein SC (1977). Am. J. Trop. Med. Hyg. Suppl, **26**: p161-

191. Griffin FM, Griffin JA, Leider JE and Silverstein SC (1975). J. Exp. Med. **142**: p1263-

192. Griffin FM, Griffin JA and Silverstein SC (1976). J. Exp. Med. **144**: p788-

193. Aikawa M, Miller LH, Johnson J and Rabbage J (1978). J. Cell Biol. **77**: p72-

194. Sinden RE (1981). Parasitological Topics (Canning EU ed). Society of protozoologists special publication No.1, Allen Press Inc., Lawrence, Kansas, USA, p242-

195. Russell DG (1983). Parasitol. **87**: p199-

196. Schwartz AL (1990). Annu. Rev. Immunol. **8**: p195-

197. Wyler DJ, Suzuki K (1983). Infect. Immun. **42**: p356-

198. Rittig MG, Bogdan C (2000). Parasitol. Today **16**: p292-

199. Allen LA, Aderem A (1996). Curr. Opin. Immunol. **8**: p36-

200. Wohnsland F, Steinmetz MO, Aebi U and Vergeres G (2000). J. Struct. Biol.**131**:p217-

201. Love DC, Kane MM, Mosser DM (1998). Exp. Parasitol. **88**: p161-

202. Mellman I (1990). Semin. Immunol. **2**: p229-

203. Geuze HJ, Slot JW and Schwartz AL (1987). J. Cell Biol. **104**: p1715-

204. Schmid SL, Fuchs R, Male P and Mellman I (1988). Cell **52**: p73-

205. Goldstein JL, Anderson RGW and Brown MS (1979). Nature **279**: p679-

206. Bray RS (1983b). J. Protozool. **30**: p322-

207. Brown MS, Anderson RGW and Goldstein JL (1983). Cell **32**: p663-

208. Alberts B, Bray D, Lewis J, Raff M, Roberts K and Watson JD (1989). Molecular Biology of the Cell. Garland Publishing Inc New York, USA, p325-

209. Shepherd VL, Konish MG and Stahl PD (1985). J. Biol. Chem, **260**: 160-

210. Clohisy DR, Bar-shavit Z, Chappel JC and Tietelbaum SL (1987), J. Biol. Chem. **262**: p15922-

211. Chung KN, Shepherd VL and Stahl PD (1984). J. Biol. Chem. **259**: p14637-

212. Bozeman PM, Hoidal JR, Shepherd VL (1988) J. Biol. Chem. **263**: p1240-

213. Mauel J (1980). Host invader interplay (Bossche HV ed). Janssen Research Foundation, Elsevier/North Holland, p165-

214. Chang KP and Dwyer DM (1978).J. Exp. Med. **142**: p515-

215. Collins HL, Schaible UE, Ernst JD, Russell DG (1997). J. Cell Sci.**110**: p191-

216. Basu N, Sett R and Das PK (1991). Biochem. J. **277**: p451-

217. Mellman IS, Plutner H, Unkeless JC, Steinman RM and Cohn ZA (1983). J. Cell. Biol. **96**: p887-

218. Sordat B and Behin R (1977). Ecologiedes Leishmanioses CNRS, INSERM, Paris, p87-

219. Chakraborty P, Sturgill-Kozycki S and Russell DG (1994). Methods in Cell Biology. **45**: p261-

220. Chang KP and Fong D (1982). Infect. Immun. **36:** p430-

221. Fong D and Chang KP (1982). Proc. NatI. Acad. Sci, USA. **79:** p7366-

222. Berg JM, Tymoczko JI, Stryer L (2001). Biochemistry. 5th ed. Freeman WH Company, USA. p395-

223. Hubbard MJ, Cohen P (1993). Trends Biochem. Sci. **18**: p172-

224. Koshland DE Jr., Goldbeter A, Stock JB (1982). Science **217**: p220-

225. Jim T, Yue L, Li J (2001). J Biol. Chem. **276**: p12879-

226. Greenberg S, Chang P, Silverstein SC (1993). J. Exp. Med. **177**: p529-

227. Greenberg S, Chang P, Wang DC, Xavier R, Seed B (1996). Proc Natl. Acad. Sci., USA. **93**: p1103-

228. Olivier M, Romero-Gallo BJ, Matte C, Blanchette J, Posner Bl, Tremblay MJ, Faure R (1998). J. Biol. Chem. **273**: p13944-

229. Brandonisio O, Panaro MA, Sisto M, Acquafredda A, Fumarola L, Leogrande D (2000). Parasitologia. **42:** p183-

230. Ghosh D, Chakraborty P (2002). Bioscience Report. **22(3-4):** p395-

231. Martiny A, Vannier-Santos MA, Borges VM, Meyer-Fernandes JR, Assreuy J, Cunha e Silva NL, deSouza W(1996). Eur. J. Cell. Biol, **71:** p206-

232. Nishizuka Y (1986). Science. **233:** p305-

233. Nishizuka Y (1988). Nature (London). **334:** p661-

234. Morel F, Doussiere J and Vignais PV (1991). Eur. J. Biochem. **91**: p523-

235. Crowley JJ and Raffin TA (1991). Am. J. Respir Cell Mol. Biol. **5**: p284

236. Yue L, Lu S, Garces J, Jin T, Li J (2000). J. Biol. Chem. **275**: p23948-

237. Olivier M, Brownsey RW and Reiner NE (1992). Proc. Natl. Acad. Sci. USA. **89**: p7481-

238. Reiner NE, NG W, Ma T, McMaster WR (1988). Proc. Natl. Acad. Sci, USA. **85**: p4330-

239. Chakraborty P, Ghosh D, Basu MK (2000) J. Biochem (Tokyo). **127**: p185-

240. Sunohara JR, Ridgway ND, Cook HW, Byers DM (2001). J. Neurochem **78**: p664-

241. Braun T, Mcllhinney RA, Vergeres G (2000). **82:** p705-

242. Thelen M, Rosen A, Nairn AC, Aderem A (1991). Nature **351**: p320-

243. Zhou X, Li J (2000). J. Biol. Chem. **275**: p20217-

244. Ramsden JJ (2000). Int. J. Biochem, Cell Biol. **32**: p475-

245. Schmitz AA, Ulrich A, Vergeres G (2000). Arch. Biochem. Biophys. **380**: p380-

246. Clark EA, Brugge JS (1995). Science **268**: p233-

247. Stefan M, Koch A, Mancini A, Mohr A, Weidner KM, Niemann H, Tamura T (2001). J. Biol. Chem **276**: p3017-

248. Reiner NE, Malemud CJ (1985). J. lmmunol. **134:** p556-

249. Baggiolini M, Wymann MP (1990). TIBS, **15**: p69-

250. Bogdan C (1998). Berl. Munch. Tierarztl. Wochenschr **111**: p409-

251. Murray HW (1984). Contemp. Top. Immunobiol. **13**: p97-

252. lyer GYN, Islam MF, Quaslel JH (1961). Nature **192**: p535-

253. Tauber AL, Babior BM (1978). Photochem. Photobiol **28**: p701-

254. Klebanoff SJ (1980). Ann. Intern. Med. **93**: p480-

255. Segal AW (1996). Mol. Med. Today **2:** p129-

256. Yu L, Quinn MT, Cross AR and Dinauer MC (1988). Proc. Natl. Acad. Sci., USA. **95**: p7993-

257. Shuhet SB, Pitt J, Bachner RL, Poplack DG (1974). Infect. Immun. **10**:p1321-

258. Hibs JB, Vavrin Z, Taintor RR (1987). J. Immunol. **138**: p550-

259. Vouldoukis I, Mureno RV, Dugas B, Ouaaz F, Bacherel PD, Moncada S and Mossalayi MD (1995). Proc. Natl. Acad. Sci, USA. **92**: p7804-

260. Moncada S and Higgs A (1993). N. Engl. J. Med. **329**: p2002-

261. Liew FY, Wei XQ, Proudfoot L (1997). Philos, Trans. R. Soc. Lond. B. Biol. Sci. **352**: p1311-

262. Hilliquin P, Borderie D, Hernvann A, Menkes CJ and Ekindjian OG (1997). Artheritis Rheum. **40**: p1512-

263. Vazquez-Torres A, Jones-Carson J and Balish E (1996). Infect. Immun. **64**: p3127-

264. Buchmuller-Rouiller Y and Mauel J (1987). Infect. Immun. **55**: p587-

265. Passwell JH, Shor R, Smolen J, Jaffe CL (1994) Int. J. Exp. Pathol. **75**: p277-

266. GIew RH, Saha AK, Das S and Remaley AT (1988). Microbiol Rev. **52**: p412-

267. Cunningham AC (2002). Exp. Mol Pathol. **72**: p132-

268. IIg T (2001). Med. Microbiol. Immunol (Berl). **190**: p13-

269. Ashford RW (1997). Ann. Trop. Med. Parasitol. **91**: p693-

270. Shaw JJ (1994). Mem. Inst. Oswaldo Cruz. **89:** p471-

271. Moore KH, Labrecque S and Matlashewski G (1993). J Immunol. **150**: p4457-

272. Evans TG, Thai L, Granger DL and Hibbs JB (Jr), (1993). J. Immunol **145**: p2662-

273. Girl OP and Singh AN (1994). Ind. Med. J. **88**: p54-

274. Plimmer HG and Thomson JD (1908). Roy Proc. Roy Soc Ser **80**: p1-

275. Murray HW (1988). Ann. Intern. Med. **108**: p595-

276. Lennartz MR, Brown EJ (1991). J. Immunol. **147**: p621-

277. Levitzki A and Gazit A (1995). Science **267**: p1782-

278. Ramazeillus C, Mishra RK, Serge ME et at. (1994). Proc. Natl. Acad. Sci., USA, **91**: p7859-

279. Powis G (1994). Pharmacol. Ther. **62**: p57-

280. Mosser DM, Vlassara H, Edelson PJ and Cerami A (1987). J.Exp. Med. **165**: p140-

281. Dutta AK, Bhaumik D and Chatterjee R (1987). J. Biol. Chem **262**: p5515-

282. Ray JC (1932). Ind. J. Med. Res. **20**: p355-

283. Russell DG, Xu S and Chakraboy P (1992). J. Cell Science, **103:** p1193-

284. Das PK, Ghosh P, Bachhawat BK and Das MK (1982). Immun. Commun.**11**: p17-

285. Dubois M, Gilles KA, Hamilton JK, Rebers PA and Smith F (1956). Analytical Chem. **28**: p350-

286. Lowry OH, Rosebrough NJ, Farr AL and Randall RJ (1951). J. Biol. Chem.**193**: p265-

287. Vlassara H, Brownlee M and Cerami A (1985). Proc. Natl. Acad. Sci., USA.**82**: p5588-

288. Hunter WM (1978). Handbook of Exp. Immunology, Weir DM (ed.) Scientific Pub. Oxford, UK, p14.4-

289. Chakraborty R, Mukherjee S, Lu HG, McGwire BS, Chang KP and Basu MK (1996). J. Parasitol. **82**: p632-

290. Mosser DM and Handman E (1992). J. Clin. Invest, **75**: p624-

291. Greenberg S, Burridge K, Silverstein SC (1990). J. Exp. Med. **172**: p1853-

292. Greeberg S, Chang P, Silverstein SC (1994). J. Biol. Chem. **269**: p3897-

293. Rosenshine I, Ruschkowski S, Foubister V, Finlay BB (1994). Infect. Immun.**62**: p4969-

294. Guan K and Dixon JE (1990). Science **249**: p553-

295. Rosenshine I, Donnenberg MS, Kaper JB, Finlay BB (1992), EMBO J **11**: p3551-

296. Ohta Y, Stossel TP, Hartwig JH (1991). Cell **67**: p275-

297. Petty HR, Todd RF (1993). J. Leukocyte Biol. **54**: p492-

298. Wang N, Butler JP, lnberg DE (1993) Science **260**: p1124-

299. Bakhiet M, Mix E, Kristensson K, Wigzell H, Olsson T (1993).Eur. J.lmmunol. **23**: p1535-

300. Li ZY, Manthey CL, Perera PY, Sher A, Vogel SN (1994). Infect. Immun. **62**: p3434-

301. Schofield L, Gerold P, Shwarz RT, Tachado S (1994). Braz. J. Med. Biol. Res. **27**: p249-

302. Akiyama T, Ogawara H (1991). Methods. Enzymol. **201**: p362-

303. Levitzki A, Gajit A, Osherov N, Posner I, Gilon C (1991). Methods. Enzymol.**201**: p347-

304. Green LC, Wagner DA, Glogwski JS, Skipper PL, Wishnok JS, Tannebaum SR (1982) Anal. Biochem.**126**: p131-

305. Gordon JA (1991), Methods. Enzymol. **201:** p477-

306. Swarup G, Cohen GS, Garbers DL (1982) Biochem. Biophys. Res. Commun. **107**: p1104-

307. Adam T, Arpin M, Prevost MC, Gounon P, Sansonetti PJ (1995). J. Cell. Biol **129**: p367-

308. Clerc P, Sansonetti PJ (1987). Infect. lmmun. **55**: p2681-

309. Clerc P, Sansonetti PJ (1988). Rouscet BF (ed), Structure and functions of the cytoskeleton. John Libbey Euro text, New York, p171-

310. James SL (1991) Exp. Parasitol. **73:** p223-

311. Nandan D, Knutson KL, Lo R, Reiner NE (2000). J. Leukoc.Biol. **67**: p464-

312. Frankenburg S, Leibovici V, Mansbach N, Turco SJ, Rosen G (1990). J. lmmunol. **145:** p4284-

313. DescoteauxA, Matlashewski G, Turco SJ (1992). J. Immunol **149**: p3008-

314. Isberg RR, G Tran Van Nhiew (1994). Trends Microbiol. **2**: p10-

315. Hanks SK, Calalb MB, Harper MC, Pakel SK (1989) Prac. Natl. Acad. Sci. USA. **89:** p8487-

316. Fisher EH, Charbonneauh H, Tonks NK (1991) Science **253**: p401-

317. Coxon PY, Summergill JJ, Ramirez JA, Miller RD (1998). Infect. Immun. **66:** p2905-

318. Finlay BB, Ruschkowski S (1991). J. Cell Sci. **99:** p283-

319. Clemens DL (1996) Trends. Microbiol. **4**: p113-

320. Holzer TJ, Nelson KE, Schauf V, Crispen RG and Anderson BR (1986) Infect. Immun. **51**: p514-

321. Clerc PL, Ryter A, Mounier J and Sansonetti P (1987). Infect. Immun. **55**: p521-

322, Tilney LG and Portnoy DA (1989). J. Cell Biol. **109**: p1597-

323. McNeely TB and Turco SJ (1990). J. Immunol. **144**: p2745-

324. Tachado SD, Gerold P, McConville MJ, Baldwin T, Quilici D, Schwerz RT and Schofield L (1996). J. Immunol. **156:** p1897-

325. Severn A, Wakelam MJO, Liew FY (1992). Biochem. Biophys. Res. Commun. **188:** p997-

326. Evans TG, Thai L, Granger DL, Hibs JB (Jr)(1993). J. lmmunol. **151**: p907-

327. Ranalay AT, Glew RH, Kuhns DB, Basford RE, Waggover AS, Grust LA and Rope M (1985). J. Biol Chem. **260**: p880-

328. Pick E (1986). Methods Enzymol. **132**: p407-

329. James SL (1991). Exp. Parasitol. **73**: p223-

330. Beverley SM and Turco SJ (1998). Trends Microbiol **6:** p35-

331. Dasgupta D, Chakraborty P and Basu MK (2000). Mol. Cell. Biochem. **209:** p1 -

332. Pimenta PF, Saraiva EM, Sacks DL (1991). Exp. Parasitol. **72:** p191-

333. Spath GF, Epstein L, Leader B, Singer SM, Avila HA, Turco SJ and Beverley SM (2000). Proc.Natl. Acad. Sci. USA. **97:** p9258-

334. McConville MJ, Turco SJ, Ferguson MA, Sacks DL (1992). EMBO J **11:** p3593-

335. IIg T (2000). EMBO J **19:** p1953-

336. McConville MJ and Homans SW (1992). J. Biol. Chem. **267:** p5855-

337. Olivier M, Baimbridge KG, Reiner NE (1992). J. Immunol. **148:** p1188-

338. Hayakawa T, Suzuki K, Suzuki S, Andrews PC, Babior BM (1986). J. Biol. Chem. **261:** p9109-

339. Stamler JS, Singel DJ, Loscaizo J (1992). Science, **258:** p1898-

340. Paul A, Pendrigh RH, Plevin R (1995). Br. J. Pharmacol. **114:** p363-

341. Proudfoot L, O'Donnell CA, Liew FY (1995). Eur J Immunol. **25:** p745-

342. McConville MJ and BlackweII JM (1991). J. Biol. Chem. **266:** p15170-

343. Tachado S, Gerold P, Schwarz R, Novakovic S, McConville M and Schofield L (1997). Proc. Natl. Acad. Sci, USA, **94:** p4022-

344. Andreev J, Borovsky Z, Rosenshine I, Rotten S (1995) FEMS Microbiol. Lett. **132**: p189-

345. Evans SW, Rennick D, Farrar WL (1987) Biochem J. **244**: p683-

346. Yamamoto M, Nishimura J, Ideguchi H, Ibayashi H (1988) Leuk. Res. **12:**p71-

347. Birkelund S, Johnsen H, Christiansen G (1994). Infect. Immun. **62**: p4900-

348. Dehio C, Prevost M, Sansonetti PJ (1995). EMBO J **11:** p2471

349. Alxinson M, Allen C, Sequeira L (1992).J. Bacteriol. **174:** p4356-

350. Allen LH, Aderem A (1995). J. Exp. Med. **182:** p829-

351. Zheleznyak A, Brown EJ (1992). J. Biol. Chem **267:** p12042-

352. Zhu Z, Bao Z, Li J (1995) J. Biol. Chem **270:** p17652-

353. Shinomiya H, Hirata H, Nakano M (1991). J. Immunol. **146**: p3617-

354. Aderem AA, Keum MM, Pure E, Cohn ZA (1986). Proc. Natl. Acad. Sci, USA. **83:** p5817-

355. Laemmli UK (1970). Nature (London) **227**: p680-

356. Bonner WM, Laskey RA (1974). Eur. J. Biochem **46**: p83-

357. Hamrick TS, Havell ES, Hortou JR, Orndorff PE (2000). Infect. Immun. **68:** p125-

358. Fernandez-Prada CM, Hoover DL, Tall BD, Hartman AB, Kopelowitz J, Venkatessan MM (2000). Infect. Immun. **68:** p3608-

359. Weied JE, Hamilton TA, Adams DO (1986). Expt. Parasitol **88:** p161-

360. Mosser DM, Handman E (1992). J. Leuk. Biol. **52**: p369-

361. Coxon PY, SummersgiII JT, Ramirez JA, Miller RD (1988). Infect. Immun. **66:** p2905-

362. Baldwin TJ, Brooks SF, Knutton S, Manjarrez-Hernandez HA, Aitken A, Williams PH (1990). Infect. Immun. **58:** p761-

363. Nishizuka Y (1984), Nature **308**: p693-

364. Corradin S, Ransijn A, Corradin G, Roggero MA, Schmitz AA, Schneider P, Mauel J, Vergeres G (1999). J. Biol. Chem. **274**: p25411-

365. Hubbard NE, Socolich RJ, Erickson KL (1996). J. Nutr. **126**: p1563-

366. Yue L, Bao Z, Li J (1999). J. Cell Physiol. **181**: p355-

367. Kraft S, Anderson WB (1983). Nature (London). **301**: p621-

368. Sturgill-Koszycki S, Schlesinger PH, Chakraborty P, Haddix PL, Collins HL, Fok AK, Allen RD, Gluck SL, Heuser J, Russel DG (1994) Science **263**: p678-

369. Benna JE, Hakim J, Labro MT (1992). Biochem. Pharmacol. **43**: p527-

370. Mochly-Rosen D (1995). Science **268**: p247-

371. Chakraborty R, Mukherjee S, Basu MK (1996). Mol. Cell Biochem. **154**: p23-

372. Rodriguez-Pena A, Rozengurt E (1984). Biochem. Biophys. Res. Commun. **120**: p1053-

373. Gresham HD, Zheleznyak A, Mormol JS, Brown EJ (1990). J. Biol. Chem. **265**: p7819-

374. Werb Z, Cohn ZA (1972), J. Biol. Chem. **247**: p2439-

375. Kitagawa S, Johnston RB (1985). J. Immunol. **135**: p3417-

376. Swanson JA (1989). J. Cell Sci. **94:** p135-

377. Novogrodsky A, Vanichkin A, Patwa M, Gazit A, Osherov N, Levitzki A (1994). Science **264**: p1319-

378. Mukherjee S, Ghosh C, Basu MK (1988), Exp. Parasitol. **66**: p18-

379. Warren GB, Houslay MD, Metcalfe JC, Birdsoll NJM (1975). Nature **258**: p684-

380. Murray HW (1982). Res. J. Reticulo. Soc. **31**: p479-

381. Young S, Parker PJ, Ullrich A, Stabel S (1987). Biochem. J. **244**: p775-

382. McNeely TB, Turco SJ (1987) Biochem. Biophys. Res. Commun. **148**: p653-

383. Castagna M, Takai Y, Kaibuchi K, Sano K, Kikkawa U, Nishizuka Y (1982). J. Biol. Chem. **257**: p7847-

384. Rossi F (1986). Biochim. Biophys. Acta. **853**: p65-

385. Chiang TM, Reizer J and Beachey EH (1989). J. Biol Chem. **264**: p2957-

386. Levitzki A (1996). Curr. Opin. Cell Biol. **8**: p239-

387. Ray M, Gam AA, Boykins AR, Kenney RT (2000). J. Infect. Dis. **181**: p1121-

388. Bray RS (1983a). J. Protozool **30**: p314-

389. Russell DG, Wilhelm H (1986). J. Immunol. **136**: p2613-

390. Dieter P (1992). FEBS Lett.**298**: p17-

391. Jalava A,Heikkila J, Lintunen M, Akerman K and Pahlman S(1992).FEBS Lett. **300**:p114-

392. Talamus P. Russell DG (1989). J. Cell Biochem.Suppl. **13E**:p158-

www.ingramcontent.com/pod-product-compliance
Lightning Source LLC
Chambersburg PA
CBHW052136170526

45162CB00003B/27